CAPSULAR STRETCHING & MAITLAND MOBILIZATION IN PERIARTHRITIS SHOULDER

Kshtrashal Singh
SUCHITRA SOLOMON J RAJA
YU CHYE WAH

CAPSULAR STRETCHING & MAITLAND MOBILIZATION IN PERIARTHRITIS SHOULDER

ELIVA PRESS

ISBN: 978-99993-4-596-5

Cover Design: Eliva Press
Cover Image: www.ingimage.com
Email: info@elivapress.com
Website: www.elivapress.com

This Eliva Press imprint is published by the registered company Eliva Press Global Ltd. part of Eliva Press S.R.L. Publishing Group

The registered company address is: Pope Hennessy Street Level 2, Hennessy Tower Port Louis, Mauritius
Eliva Press S.R.L. Publishing Group legal address is: Bd. Cuza-Voda 1/4 of. 21, Chisinau, Moldova, Europe

THE EFFECTIVENESS OF MODIFIED POSTERIOR CAPSULAR STRETCHING VS GRADE 3 MAITLAND MOBILIZATION AMONG PATIENTS WITH PERIARTHRITIS SHOULDER. A QUASI EXPERIMENTAL STUDY

INTRODUCTION

1.1 Background of the study

Musculoskeletal disorders (MSDs) include a variety of conditions that impact the joints bones and muscles often manifesting as pain and injury in these areas. Upper limb musculoskeletal disorders (ULMSDs) have emerged as a significant global health concern, particularly among healthcare workers. These disorders are characterized by their multifactorial etiology, involving physical and psychosocial risk factors. Clinical laboratory workers in the healthcare sector, especially those who frequently use microscopes, face an elevated risk of developing ULMSDs. Their work exposes them to prolonged static muscular activity, which can lead to disorders affecting the neck, shoulders, and upper extremities. Various work-related psychosocial elements, such as high job demands workplace stress, lack of social support, and time pressures, compound this occupational hazard. The prevalence of ULMSDs among healthcare workers, particularly those in laboratory settings, is alarmingly high. Research has shown that many professionals experience musculoskeletal pain, with the neck and shoulders most commonly affected areas. For instance, a study by Forouzan (2015) revealed that 82.8% of subjects were at high risk of developing MSDs, with 55.9% reporting neck pain and 43.8% experiencing shoulder pain. Moreover, 68.9% of the participants had experienced some form of musculoskeletal pain within the past year. Several factors contribute to the development of ULMSDs among laboratory workers. These include the duration of daily work hours, the number of patients or samples processed, and the ergonomic design of workstations. Interestingly, while factors such as body mass index (BMI) and years of experience were not significantly associated with pain in some studies, the relationship between musculoskeletal pain and work-related factors like daily work hours and workload was significant. The high prevalence of ULMSDs among laboratory workers, particularly those using microscopes, underscores the need for targeted interventions. These may include ergonomic improvements in workstation design, implementation of regular break schedules to reduce prolonged static postures, and addressing psychosocial factors in the workplace. Additionally, raising awareness about proper posture and techniques for microscope use could mitigate the risk of developing these disorders. In conclusion, ULMSDs represent a significant occupational health challenge in the healthcare sector, especially among laboratory workers. The multifactorial nature of these disorders, involving both physical and psychosocial elements, necessitates a comprehensive approach to prevention and management. Addressing workplace ergonomics, work organization, and psychosocial factors may reduce the prevalence and impact of ULMSDs among this vulnerable occupational group. Osmani & Farhadi Hassankiadeh, (2020)

Healthcare providers frequently encounter patients with musculoskeletal shoulder discomfort. While conservative treatments have demonstrated efficacy in alleviating symptoms and improving functional outcomes, a substantial proportion of patients continue to experience discomfl01ort over extended periods. Despite the implementation of conservative measures, research indicates that a considerable portion of patients—approximately 40%—continue to report shoulder discomfort one year after initial presentation, with half still experiencing symptoms after six months. This persistence of symptoms underscores the complexity and challenges of managing shoulder pain effectively. One of the critical dilemmas in understanding and managing shoulder pain lies in the ambiguous nature of its underlying pathophysiology. Shoulder pain can arise from many factors, and its aetiology may involve both peripheral and central pain pathways. Peripheral mechanisms encompass structural abnormalities within the shoulder joint, such as rotator cuff injuries, tendonitis, or bursitis. In contrast, central mechanisms involve alterations in the processing of pain signals within the central nervous system. The debate surrounding the contribution of peripheral versus central mechanisms to shoulder pain underscores the need for a comprehensive and multifaceted approach to its assessment and management. By recognizing the potential involvement of peripheral and central pain pathways, healthcare practitioners can tailor treatment strategies to address the underlying mechanisms contributing to a patient's symptoms. Persistent shoulder pain poses a significant concern for healthcare providers due to its potential impact on patient's quality of life and functional abilities. Chronic pain conditions can significantly impair patients' physical and psychological well-being, leading to disability, decreased mobility, and diminished overall health outcomes. Moreover, persistent shoulder pain raises important clinical considerations regarding its management. Healthcare practitioners must carefully evaluate patients presenting with chronic shoulder pain to identify any underlying contributing factors, such as concurrent medical conditions, psychosocial stressors, or maladaptive pain processing mechanisms. Addressing persistent shoulder pain requires a holistic approach that incorporates pharmacological and non-pharmacological interventions to alleviate symptoms, improve function, and enhance patients' overall well-being. In addition to traditional pain management modalities, such as nonsteroidal anti-inflammatory drugs (NSAIDs), physical therapy, and corticosteroid injections, emerging treatments targeting central pain processing pathways, such as cognitive-behavioral therapy (CBT) and mindfulness-based interventions, hold promise in the management of chronic shoulder pain. Furthermore, patient education and self-management strategies are crucial in empowering individuals to participate in their care and optimize treatment outcomes actively. By fostering collaborative partnerships between healthcare providers and patients, tailored treatment plans can be developed to address the multifaceted nature of persistent shoulder pain, ultimately improving patients' quality of life and functional status. Haik et al. (2019)

Shoulder discomfort and dysfunction often manifest as common symptoms of periarthritis. This condition primarily arises from inflammatory lesions affecting various structures surrounding the shoulder joint, such as the joint capsule, ligaments, bursa, tendons, and muscles. Additionally, degenerative changes within the shoulder joint itself can contribute to its onset. In severe cases, peri arthritis can lead to limited mobility of the shoulder joint and muscle atrophy. The overarching goals of therapy aim to alleviate paralysis and pain, alleviate symptoms, and restore functional activity. This therapeutic approach encompasses addressing a multitude of factors, both internal and environmental, that contribute to the pathophysiological processes underlying periarthritis. Zhaohong Zeng et al. (2022)

Periarthritis of the shoulder is a condition that leads to significant pain and a widespread limitation in both active and passive movement of the glenohumeral joint, particularly affecting shoulder abduction and external rotation. This condition affects 3% to 5% of the overall population, with its incidence rising to as much as 20% among individuals with diabetes. Its prevalence ranges between 2% and 5%. It predominantly occurs in females, most frequently within the age group of 40 to 60 years, and is ten times more likely to affect those with diabetes. Agrawal et al. (2019)

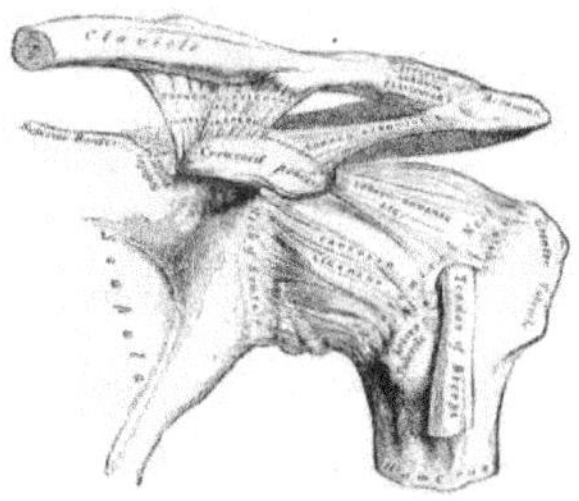

Miniato MA, Anand P, Varacallo M. (2024)

Fig 1 Shoulder anatomy

1.2 Anatomy of shoulder joint

The shoulder is an intricate and adaptable part of the human body, largely due to the sophisticated articulation of the glenohumeral joint, which provides a vast range of motion. This joint is crucial for connecting the upper limb to the torso through the sternoclavicular joint, a synovial joint. The shoulder girdle is composed of the scapula and clavicle, which join with the proximal humerus of the upper limb. The shoulder includes four primary joints: the glenohumeral, scapulothoracic, acromioclavicular (AC) and sternoclavicular (SC). The acromioclavicular joint links the clavicle to the acromion of the scapula, while the sternoclavicular joint connects the upper limb to the central body structure. The scapulothoracic joint, which allows the scapula to glide over the back of the thoracic cage, functions more as a sliding area than a true joint. The glenohumeral joint, a highly flexible ball-and-socket synovial joint, is supported by the tendons of the rotator cuff and the biceps and triceps brachii muscles. This joint can perform various movements, including abduction, adduction, flexion, extension, internal and external rotation, and horizontal adduction and abduction. These movements contribute to the shoulder's stability and protect it from injuries and dislocations. A fibrocartilaginous ring called the labrum also deepens the joint socket, further enhancing its stability. The primary blood vessel supplying the shoulder area is the axillary artery, which branches out to nourish the region through several arteries, including the anterior and posterior humeral circumflex arteries, subscapular artery, thoracoacromial artery, lateral thoracic artery, and superior thoracic artery. Before becoming the axillary artery past the first rib's lateral margin, the subclavian artery provides branches that supply the shoulder. The thyrocervical trunk, branching from the subclavian artery, contributes to this network through the suprascapular and transverse cervical arteries. Occasionally, the dorsal scapular artery also branches from the subclavian or transverse cervical artery. The shoulder's intrinsic muscles facilitate various movements by linking the scapula and clavicle to the humerus. The deltoid muscle, for example, enables flexion and medial rotation (anterior aspect), arm abduction (middle aspect), and lateral rotation and extension of the arm (posterior aspect). These muscles are innervated by specific nerves and contribute to the shoulder's stability and motion. Additional muscles play crucial roles in shoulder joint movement. The trapezius aids in raising, rotating, and retracting the scapula, depending on the activated fibre section. The latissimus dorsi extends, adducts, and medially rotates the upper limb. The levator scapulae elevate the scapula while the rhomboids rotate and retract it. The anterior serratus is essential for positioning the scapula against the thoracic wall, enabling rotation and arm abduction. The major and minor pectoralis muscles contribute to arm adduction, with the major also flexing the clavicle and the minor protracting the scapula and depressing the shoulder. The subclavius assists in clavicle stability, and the coracobrachialis facilitates arm flexion and adduction. Lastly, the biceps brachii prevent shoulder dislocation, flex the forearm, and supinate the forearm, while the triceps brachii avoid shoulder dislocation and act as a significant extensor muscle of the forearm. These muscles, innervated by specific nerves, work together to ensure the shoulder's functional and structural integrity. Miniato MA, Anand P, Varacallo M. (2024)

1.3 Biomechanics of Shoulder Joint

The interaction of the glenohumeral, acromioclavicular, scapulothoracic, and sternoclavicular joints governs the shoulder's complex biomechanics. As the most mobile joint in the human body, the glenohumeral joint affords the hand a wide range of positions, though this mobility also introduces challenges and potential instability. The presence of 18 muscles working in synergy makes precise kinematic analyses and clinical assessments particularly difficult. Being dynamic and not weight-bearing, the glenohumeral joint is prone to substantial changes in both skeletal and muscular structures, alongside common tendon overuse. Each anatomical component must work together seamlessly for the shoulder to operate effectively as a functional unit. Signals from the central nervous system prompt the muscle-tendon unit to generate tension, which is then applied through the tendon acting as a lever arm on the joint. A stable fulcrum, essential for efficiency, is provided by a combination of static and dynamic factors, including the joint capsule, ligaments, and the shape of bones. However, evaluating biomechanically significant features in a living body without using invasive methods, such as measuring joint reaction forces, remains challenging. Goetti et al. (2020)

Exploring the glenohumeral joint with this framework could illuminate the mechanics of upper limb movement. Predicting muscle function involves estimating the forces generated by muscles, which requires understanding their coactivation. Electromyography (EMG) and musculoskeletal modelling offer insights, yet they must reveal clear relationships between muscle load and activation. Furthermore, despite higher muscle activation levels, no significant impact of load on the risk of glenohumeral joint dislocation was observed based on the time spent above a critical shear-compression ratio. This gap in findings may be due to local variations within the glenohumeral joint itself. Fatigue in the shoulder can lead to changes in the kinematics of the elbow, trunk, and shoulder during precision tasks. The absence of significant changes in muscle activation and the minimal influence of load on dislocation risk could be better understood by examining the adaptations in the muscle function of the glenohumeral joint. Assila et al (2021)

1.4 Epidemiology

Periarthritis of shoulder is a common and debilitating shoulder condition characterized by progressive pain and loss of passive and active range of motion in the shoulder joint. The epidemiology of periarthritis of shoulder is not fully understood, but some key points: Incidence: The one-year prevalence rate of periarthritis of shoulder is estimated to be around 0.35% among adults aged 65 and older in the United States, translating to approximately 142,000 older adults affected. The overall incidence in the general population is estimated to be 2-5%. Periarthritis of shoulder is more common in women than men with some studies reporting 59-70% prevalence in women. It typically affects individuals between 40-60 years of age. Risk factors: Diabetes and Parkinson's disease have been identified as significant risk factors for developing periarthritis of shoulder in the elderly. Other potential risk factors include a sedentary lifestyle, systemic inflammation, and oxidative stress. Some studies have suggested a slight seasonal trend, with more cases occurring from August through December, but a clear seasonal pattern has yet to be firmly established. The specific triggers for primary (idiopathic) periarthritis of shoulder remain elusive. Potential triggers that have been investigated include certain medications, infections, and traumas, but the evidence is inconclusive. In summary, periarthritis shoulder is a relatively common condition that disproportionately affects middle-aged and older women, with diabetes and Parkinson's disease being significant risk factors. Further research is needed to fully elucidate the epidemiology and underlying causes of this debilitating shoulder disorder. De La Serna et al. (2021)

1.5 Occupational Interactions with Periarthritis Shoulder

Manual handling tasks that involve heavy lifting, pushing, pulling, holding, or carrying can significantly increase the risk of developing shoulder disorders, including periarthritis of the shoulder. Working with the arms raised above shoulder height, performing repetitive work, being exposed to vibration, and adopting awkward postures are all associated with a higher incidence of periarthritis shoulder. In addition to physical factors, psychosocial job demands and stress have also been linked to an increased risk of developing periarthritis shoulder. This highlights the importance of addressing workplace physical and psychosocial risk factors to prevent and manage this condition effectively. Early structured physiotherapy and exercise programs designed to increase physical capacity have shown promising results in managing periarthritis of shoulders in the workplace. These interventions typically include supervised exercises, manual therapy techniques, and a progressive home exercise program to improve shoulder mobility and strength. To comprehensively prevent and manage periarthritis shoulder, workplace interventions that target multiple risk factors, such as ergonomic modifications, job rotation, and stress management, are recommended. Ergonomic interventions may include adjusting workstation layout, providing mechanical aids, and modifying work methods to reduce exposure to high-risk tasks. When evaluating the effectiveness of medical and surgical interventions for periarthritis shoulder, it is crucial to include workplace outcomes in clinical trials. Assessing factors such as return to work, work performance, and job satisfaction can provide valuable insights into how well these interventions translate to real-world occupational settings. In conclusion, a multifaceted approach that addresses both physical and psychosocial risk factors in the workplace is essential for preventing and managing periarthritis shoulder. Early structured physiotherapy, exercise programs, and ergonomic interventions have shown promise in managing this condition. Future research should incorporate workplace outcomes to understand better the effectiveness of medical and surgical interventions in an occupational context. Chan et al. (2017)

1.6 Aetiology & Risk Factor

Periarthritis of the shoulder, also known as primary or idiopathic periarthritis, is a condition with an unclear cause. When this disorder is linked to specific traumas or systemic health issues, such as Type II diabetes mellitus, thyroid disorders, rheumatoid arthritis and others, it is classified as secondary periarthritis of the shoulder. This distinction is crucial for understanding the underlying factors and appropriate treatment approaches. The condition is relatively common, with an estimated incidence rate of 3% to 5% in the general population. However, it shows a higher prevalence among specific demographics. Notably, it predominantly affects women and is most prevalent in individuals aged between 40 and 60 years. This age group is particularly susceptible, possibly due to age-related degenerative processes in the shoulder joint and surrounding tissues. Moreover, individuals with diabetes mellitus are at a significantly increased risk. The incidence of periarthritis of the shoulder in the diabetic population is as high as 20%. This elevated risk can be attributed to the systemic effects of diabetes, which can lead to changes in connective tissue and reduced blood flow, thereby increasing the vulnerability to musculoskeletal disorders like periarthritis. Understanding these distinctions and epidemiological data is essential for healthcare providers. It aids in the accurate diagnosis and tailored management of periarthritis, whether primary or secondary. Effective treatment and management strategies can significantly improve the quality of life for those affected by this painful and potentially debilitating condition. Cavalleri et al., (2020)

Diabetes encompasses a group of chronic conditions characterized by elevated blood sugar levels, with type 1 and type 2 diabetes being the most common forms, accounting for 8% and 90% of cases, respectively. While the cardiovascular, ocular, neurological, and renal complications of diabetes are widely recognized, its musculoskeletal effects often receive less attention. Musculoskeletal issues like a frozen shoulder can significantly impact a patient's quality of life and deserve greater consideration. Frozen shoulder, in particular, has been linked to diabetes, with theories suggesting that glycation processes or inflammatory responses may lead to capsular fibrosis and subsequent joint contracture. To establish a potential causal relationship between diabetes and frozen shoulder, it's crucial to understand their temporal association. This requires evidence from longitudinal observational studies that can elucidate the sequence of events and potential mechanisms linking these two conditions. Investigating this relationship lies in its implications for patient care and management. If diabetes is indeed a contributing factor to frozen shoulder, early intervention and targeted treatments could potentially prevent or mitigate this painful condition in diabetic patients. Moreover, understanding this connection could improve screening protocols and earlier detection of musculoskeletal complications in individuals with diabetes. By focusing on the temporal aspect, researchers aim to determine whether the onset of diabetes precedes the development of a frozen shoulder, strengthening the case for a causal link. This information could be valuable for healthcare providers in developing comprehensive care plans that address both the metabolic and musculoskeletal aspects of diabetes management. In conclusion, while diabetes is commonly associated with various systemic complications, its potential role in musculoskeletal conditions like frozen shoulder warrants further investigation. Longitudinal studies examining the temporal relationship between these conditions are essential for advancing our understanding and improving patient outcomes. Dyer et al. (2023)

1.7 Sign and Symptoms

Periarthritis of the shoulder is a condition that progresses through several distinct phases, each characterized by specific symptoms and histological changes. The initial phase often called the painful phase, is marked by significant pain and a progressive restriction of shoulder movement. During this phase, hypertrophic synovitis with hypervascularity is observed, although the capsular tissue appears normal. This stage can be particularly debilitating, as the pain is often severe and can interfere with daily activities and sleep. Following the painful phase is the 'freezing' stage, which typically lasts around nine months. During this period, symptoms gradually worsen, and histological examinations reveal perivascular synovitis and collagen deposition. The shoulder becomes increasingly stiff, and the range of motion significantly reduces. This stage is crucial as the inflammatory process continues, forming scar tissue within the joint capsule. The subsequent phase is known as the 'frozen' phase, lasting one to four months. In this stage, stiffness becomes the predominant symptom, overshadowing pain. The shoulder joint's movement is severely restricted due to the dense collagenous tissue within the capsule. This phase is often the most challenging for patients, as the limited mobility can severely impact their ability to perform everyday tasks. Finally, the 'thawing' phase occurs, gradually resolving symptoms. The duration of this phase is highly variable, ranging from a few months to up to two years. During this time, the shoulder's range of motion slowly improves as the scar tissue remodels and the inflammation subsides. However, the extent of recovery can vary significantly among individuals, with some patients experiencing residual stiffness and pain even after the thawing phase. The clinical presentation of periarthritis of the shoulder does not always follow a strict stepwise progression, and there can be significant variation in how the condition manifests and resolves. Diagnosis is primarily clinical, with pain and stiffness being the hallmark symptoms. The onset of pain is usually gradual, developing over several months, and is often accompanied by night pain, which can disrupt sleep. The pain is typically described as a deep ache, sometimes poorly localized, and may radiate to the deltoid origin or the biceps area. Physical examination findings in periarthritis are often nonspecific. There are usually no point tenderness and rotator cuff strength remain normal. However, both passive and active ranges of motion (ROM) are globally reduced, which is best assessed through passive external rotation with the arm by the side. Laboratory tests are generally normal but can be useful in identifying underlying conditions such as diabetes or thyroid disease, which are associated with an increased risk of developing periarthritis. Imaging studies play a limited role in the diagnosis of periarthritis. Plain radiographs of the shoulder are typically normal but can help exclude other conditions such as calcific tendinopathy, glenohumeral arthritis, acromioclavicular arthritis, or shoulder dislocation. In cases of calcific tendinopathy, disuse osteopenia may be visible on radiographs. Advanced imaging modalities such as arthrography, technetium bone scans, and magnetic resonance imaging (MRI) are not routinely indicated for evaluating adhesive capsulitis. Still, they can be useful in ruling out other pathologies. Date and Rahman (2020)

1.8 Pathophysiology

The pathophysiology of periarthritis shoulder, involves a complex interplay of inflammatory and fibrotic processes within the shoulder joint capsule. In the inflammatory Phase, synovial inflammation is a crucial initiating event characterized by infiltrating inflammatory cells (lymphocytes, mast cells) and releasing inflammatory mediators (cytokines, interleukins). Moreover, elevated levels of pro-inflammatory cytokines (IL-1β, IL-6, TNF-α) and growth factors (TGF-β, PDGF) contribute to the inflammatory cascade and subsequent fibrosis. Furthermore, oxidative stress and the formation of advanced glycation end-products (AGEs) may play a role, particularly in patients with diabetes, leading to increased inflammation and fibrosis. The second Phase is fibrotic; in this phase, the fibroblast proliferation and differentiation into myofibroblasts occur within the joint capsule, particularly in the rotator interval and anterosuperior regions. Plus, Myofibroblasts produce excessive amounts of collagen and other extracellular matrix proteins, leading to capsular thickening and contracture. Also, its increased expression of matrix metalloproteinases (MMPs) and tissue inhibitors of metalloproteinases (TIMPs) contribute to the dysregulation of matrix remodeling. The neo-angiogenesis and nerve growth factor (NGF) expression may also contribute to pain and stiffness. The final is the pathological changes, where the joint capsule becomes thickened, inflamed, and contracted, particularly in the anterosuperior and rotator interval regions. The coracohumeral ligament and rotator interval also exhibit thickening and fibrosis. Histologically, the capsule shows dense collagen deposition, increased myofibroblast population, and inflammatory cell infiltration. The Potential Mechanisms, genetic predisposition, hormonal factors, and metabolic disorders (e.g., diabetes, thyroid dysfunction) may contribute to the development of a periarthritis of shoulder. Immobilization or trauma may also trigger the inflammatory cascade and subsequent fibrosis. Finally, the autoimmune mechanisms and molecular mimicry have been proposed but require further investigation. Kraal et al. (2020)

1.9 History & Physical Examination

Based on a study by Somerville et al. (2017), musculoskeletal disorders are the most common chronic health issue in Canada, causing the most disability and utilizing the most healthcare resources. Shoulder complaints are the third most prevalent musculoskeletal problem, with many patients being referred to orthopaedic surgery or primary care sports medicine clinics for knee issues. Diagnosing shoulder pain and disability can be challenging for physicians due to the various causes and potential for multiple disorders in the same patient. A thorough patient history, clinical evaluation of the entire shoulder area, and clinical tests and imaging may be necessary for an accurate diagnosis. However, even with these measures, misdiagnosis can occur, and more invasive tests like MRI and arthroscopic exams are often required. Despite the importance of these diagnostic tools, patient history can be sufficient to predict shoulder pathologies. Research has shown that a diagnosis can be made with history alone. For example, studies have found that the history led to a correct diagnosis in 83% and 76% of general medical outpatients. Similarly, symptoms like age over 65, night pain, and sudden onset of pain can predict specific shoulder conditions like rotator cuff tears and SLAP lesions. However, primary care physicians often refer musculoskeletal conditions to orthopaedic surgeons when nonsurgical intervention is more appropriate. This can reduce the efficiency of these services and affect the quality of care. Applying a similar approach to shoulder care could streamline patient care, reduce referrals for further diagnostic tests, and improve the efficiency of these services.

1.9.1 Different Diagnosis

Periarthritis of shoulder, is a condition that often comes into the diagnostic picture regarding shoulder pain and restricted mobility. However, it's crucial to approach this condition with a discerning eye, as several other shoulder pathologies can mimic its symptoms. Arriving at an accurate diagnosis involves meticulously evaluating various factors, including medical history, physical examination, and strategic utilization of diagnostic imaging techniques. The differential diagnosis for periarthritis of shoulder encompasses various potential culprits, each with unique characteristics and implications. Cervical radiculopathy, a condition involving nerve root compression in the neck, can manifest with similar symptoms of pain and restricted range of motion. Rotator cuff tendinopathy, an inflammation or degeneration of the tendons that stabilize the shoulder joint, is another contender that must be considered. Glenohumeral osteoarthritis, a degenerative joint disease affecting the shoulder, can also present with overlapping symptoms, further complicating the diagnostic process. Hill (2024)

Diagnostic imaging plays a pivotal role in this intricate puzzle, not necessarily to confirm periarthritis of shoulder but to rule out concurrent pathologies contributing to the patient's symptoms. Plain radiographs, or X-rays, are valuable for excluding conditions such as tumours, osteoarthritis, and fractures. Ultrasound and magnetic resonance imaging (MRI) can provide:

- Deeper insights.
- Revealing potential rotator cuff tears.

- Biceps tendon disorders.
- Joint effusions (fluid accumulation).

However, it's important to note that no single imaging modality can definitively diagnose periarthritis of shoulder. While suggestive, findings like the thickening of the coracohumeral ligament or joint capsule are not specific to this condition alone. A recent study by Tran et al. employed latent class analysis on ultrasound findings to identify distinct clusters of shoulder pathology, highlighting the potential limitations of traditional patho-anatomical classifications in capturing the full complexity of shoulder conditions. In addition to imaging techniques, the "lidocaine test," involving a subacromial injection, can aid in establishing the diagnosis of periarthritis of shoulder. This diagnostic procedure can provide valuable insights into the underlying cause of the patient's symptoms by temporarily alleviating pain and improving the range of motion. Ultimately, diagnosing periarthritis of shoulder remains a clinical endeavour, relying on a comprehensive evaluation of the patient's medical history, a thorough physical examination, and a strategic approach to ruling out other potential causes through imaging and diagnostic tests. It's a process that requires a keen eye for detail, a deep understanding of shoulder pathologies, and a willingness to explore the complexities beneath the surface of this enigmatic condition. Walker-Bone and Van Der Windt (2021)

1.9.2 Special Test

The restriction of shoulder range of motion (ROM) is a common issue associated with various shoulder injuries. This limitation often results from tight muscles surrounding the shoulder joint and the glenohumeral (GH) joint capsule. Research indicates that restricted GH internal rotation (IR) ROM, caused by tightness in the posterior shoulder tissues, can lead to shoulder impingement and labrum lesions. Additionally, tightness in these tissues can cause the humeral head to move anteriorly during GH horizontal adduction (HA), resulting in abnormal arthrokinematics of the GH joint. To diagnose the causes of shoulder injuries, clinicians frequently measure GH IR and HA passive ROM (PROM). These measurements are typically conducted with the patient in a supine position, ensuring the scapula is fixed to achieve accurate results. Similarly, GH HA PROM is measured by stabilizing the scapular lateral border to prevent unnecessary scapular movement. Although these methods facilitate precise measurement of shoulder ROM, the results can vary depending on the examiner's expertise. Another method for assessing combined shoulder IR ROM is the scratch test. During this test, both hands are placed on the upper and lower regions of the back, respectively, to measure combined shoulder IR, adduction, and extension on the lower arm side. This maneuver is advantageous as it quickly and easily identifies limitations in shoulder movement. Various stretching exercises, such as sleeper and cross-body stretches, are commonly employed in clinical settings to address posterior shoulder tightness. Previous studies have demonstrated that GH IR and HA ROM significantly increase after these stretching exercises, supporting the validity of GH IR and HA PROM as indicators of posterior shoulder tightness. However, traditional methods of measuring GH IR and HA PROM can take time and effort. Although the scratch test can quickly identify combined GH IR ROM, no study has examined the relationship between the scratch test and GH IR and HA ROM. Previous research has only identified a significant correlation between GH IR and HA PROM. This study investigates the relationship between the scratch test, GH IR, and HA ROM. The scratch test is widely used in clinical settings to identify limitations in combined shoulder movements. Still, its correlation with GH IR and HA ROM has yet to be thoroughly examined. This study aims to fill this gap by exploring the relationship between these measurements. In total, 24 university students without shoulder pain participated in this study. GH IR ROM was passively measured supine with 90° of shoulder and elbow flexion on the tested side. An examiner passively lowered the forearm for GH IR while gripping the coracoid process to identify scapular movement. When the scapular movement was detected, passive IR was stopped, and a smartphone was placed on the dorsal side of the forearm to measure the end-range GH IR angle using an inclinometer application. To measure GH HA PROM, participants were positioned supine with 90° of shoulder and elbow flexion on the tested side. An examiner fixed the lateral border of the scapula using the thenar eminence to limit unnecessary scapular protraction while moving the humerus across the body without humeral rotation. A smartphone was placed on the dorsal side of the humerus at the end range of GH HA, and the HA angle was measured using the inclinometer application. During the scratch test, participants placed one hand on the lower region of the back and the other on the upper area of the back. The distance between the two fists was measured using a tape measure. Measurements were performed in a random order, with bilateral measures repeated three times. The mean value of the three measurements was used for data analysis. The study found a significant correlation between the scratch test, GH IR, and HA PROM. Specifically, the scratch test showed a moderate to good correlation with GH HA PROM and a fair correlation with GH IR PROM. These findings suggest that the scratch test could be a helpful and quick method for identifying GH joint ROM limitations. In conclusion, the scratch test demonstrates a significant relationship with GH IR and HA PROM, indicating its potential as a quick and effective tool for assessing shoulder ROM limitations. Further research should include subjects of various ages and those with shoulder pain to validate these findings across different populations. Kang (2018)

Procedure of Apley's Scratch, Almoallim et al. (2021)

- Patient position:

  High sitting

- Hand placement:

To stabilize the scapula and ensure isolated glenohumeral (GH) joint movement without scapular elevation, place the right hand firmly on the right shoulder over the acromioclavicular (AC) joint. On the other hand, hold the proximal forearm and perform shoulder abduction up to 90 degrees, ensuring pure GH joint movement without scapular elevation. At this point, there should be no scapular elevation. While maintaining shoulder abduction at 90 degrees, perform external rotation (ER) and internal rotation (IR). Next, adduct the shoulder back to the zero position, where the forearm and elbow are beside the body, and then perform shoulder extension. After completing these steps, remove the right hand from the right shoulder and proceed with forward flexion. Subsequently, the ER and IR should be assessed with the arms at the sides at zero abduction. Repeat the same approach for the left shoulder, using the left hand to stabilize the scapula over the left AC joint. This systematic approach ensures that each movement is isolated to the GH joint, preventing compensatory movements from the scapula. For shoulder abduction, hold the proximal forearm and raise the arm to 90 degrees. This movement should be from the GH joint, with no scapular elevation. This isolation ensures that the movement is accurately assessed and performed without compensatory actions from the scapula. While the shoulder is abducted at 90 degrees, perform ER and IR to evaluate the range of motion and identify any limitations or discomfort. After assessing the ER and IR at 90 degrees abduction, the shoulder is adducted back to zero. In this position, the forearm and elbow should be beside the body. From here, shoulder extension is performed to evaluate the posterior shoulder's flexibility and strength. This movement is crucial for reaching behind or extending the arm backward. Next, take off the right hand from the right shoulder and proceed with forward flexion. This movement involves raising the arm before the body and assessing the anterior shoulder's flexibility and strength. Forward flexion is essential for activities that involve reaching forward or overhead. Finally, the ER and IR should be assessed with the arms at the sides at zero abduction. This position allows for a neutral assessment of the shoulder's rotational capabilities without the influence of kidnapping. By evaluating ER and IR in this position, we can easily identify any limitations or discomfort that may not be apparent in other positions. Repeat the same approach for the left shoulder, using your left hand to stabilize the scapula over the left AC joint. This ensures that both shoulders are assessed and treated equally, comprehensively evaluating shoulder movement and stability.

- Interpretation

A positive Apley's scratch test suggests possible rotator cuff issues, capsular tightness, or shoulder periarthritis. Though it doesn't pinpoint a specific condition, it indicates a general loss of functional range of motion. The test should be conducted on both shoulders for comparison, as the non-dominant side may naturally show slightly more restriction. Batool et al. (2016)

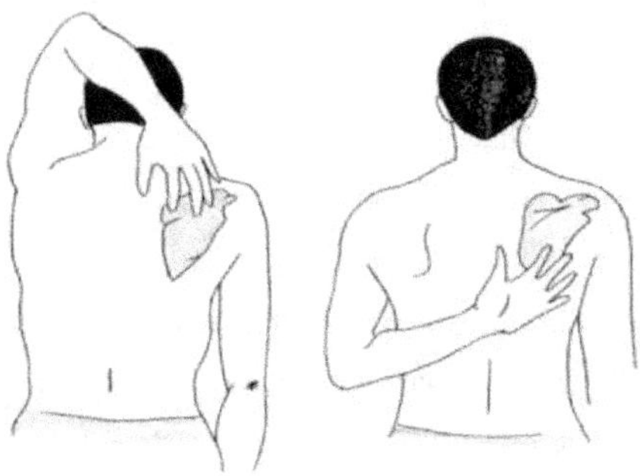

Fig. 2 Apley's scratch

1.10 Medical Management

The medical management of periarthritis shoulder, centres on non-surgical approaches designed to lessen pain and enhance joint flexibility. This medical regimen combines drug-based treatments and occasionally, injectable therapies to address the rigidity and discomfort associated with the condition. (Maya, 2017)

Nonsteroidal anti-inflammatory drugs (NSAIDs) like ibuprofen and naproxen are commonly used to treat the pain and inflammation linked with peri arthritis shoulder. These drugs are particularly useful in the early, painful stages. For cases that present with more intense symptoms, a short course of oral corticosteroids may be prescribed to reduce inflammation quickly. Research, including studies compiled in medical databases such as PubMed, supports the use of NSAIDs in managing the symptoms associated with this disorder. Furthermore, targeted intra-articular corticosteroid injections provide another critical component of periarthritis shoulder treatment. Administering these injections directly into the shoulder joint can lead to rapid pain alleviation and mobility enhancement. Literature reviews reveal that when corticosteroid injections are used alongside physical therapy, patients report significant improvements in pain relief and functional ability compared to those undergoing physical therapy alone. Moreover, hydrodilatation is an additional treatment modality for peri arthritis shoulder. This intervention entails injecting sterile saline, corticosteroids, and local anaesthetics into the joint capsule to stretch and reduce adhesions. Clinical evidence has demonstrated that hydrodilatation can improve joint movement range and alleviate pain in individuals with periarthritis of shoulder. It is paramount to educate patients about the periarthritis shoulder and emphasize their role in the treatment process. Understanding the condition and committing to regular stretching and strengthening activities can help retain joint mobility and stave off subsequent rigidity. Challoumas et al., (2020)

To sum up, the medical management of periarthritis shoulder is a comprehensive strategy that leverages drug treatments, injection therapies, and exercise to combat the various manifestations of the condition. The treatment choice is tailored to the patient's specific symptoms and disease phase, striving to mitigate pain, boost functionality, and rejuvenate joint movement. Clinical trials and systematic reviews continually validate the success of these treatment options, offering a solid empirical foundation for contemporary medical techniques. (Maya, 2017)

1.11 Physiotherapy Management

The rehabilitation strategy for periarthritis of the shoulder is a vital facet of the healing framework for this incapacitating ailment. The disorder is marked by a trifecta of symptoms: pain, stiffness, and a restricted range of motion within the shoulder joint. Clinically, the condition advances through three distinct phases: the freezing phase marks the onset of augmenting discomfort with a downtrend in mobility; the frozen phase is characterized by stabilizing pain levels, albeit with augmented stiffness; and finally, the thawing phase witnesses a gradual resurgence of shoulder mobility. Physiotherapeutic Approach to Pain Alleviation: Addressing pain is foundational, enhancing the acceptance and execution of additional therapy measures. Cold packs, heat applications, and transcutaneous electrical nerve stimulation are methods that assist in managing pain. While NSAIDs are prevalent for their pain and inflammation management properties, vigilant monitoring is required due to their potential adverse effects. In the initial treatment phase, it is essential to perform gentle exercises aimed at preserving joint motion to the greatest extent without triggering additional pain. This involves passive exercises, wherein the therapist assists the arm's movement, and active-assistive exercises that involve the patient's effort in concert with aid. (Kolathuru et al., 2023)

As patients transition into the frozen phase, the emphasis shifts to more rigorous stretching and the application of joint mobilizations. These techniques, including hands-on therapy such as joint manipulation by the physical therapist, aim to elongate the joint capsule and alleviate tissue stiffness, thereby improving flexibility. Progressing into and especially during the thawing phase, building muscle strength becomes a central theme of therapy. Augmenting the strength of shoulder-surrounding muscles, notably the rotator cuff and scapular stabilizers, fosters joint stability and facilitates normal functioning. Such exercises are tailored to fortify these key muscle groups. Patient enlightenment on the condition's progression and nature is key to setting realistic expectations and fostering treatment plan adherence. Additionally, patients are equipped with self-help techniques and at-home exercises, which are imperative for the enduring management and deterrence of symptom reoccurrence. Physiotherapy incorporates assorted modalities like ultrasound therapy, laser treatment, and shortwave diathermy to alleviate pain and inflammation, although individual responses can dictate their applicability and effectiveness. (Mezian & Chang, 2019)

1.12 Literature Review

1.12.1 Periarthritis of shoulder

Somaiya et al. (2021) stated that, this study explores the comparative effectiveness of two physical therapy interventions, namely the Muscle Energy Technique (MET) and the Kalternborn Mobilisation Technique, on alleviating pain in diabetic individuals afflicted with Periarthritis of the Shoulder. This condition, known as periarthritis of shoulder, affects approximately 11-30% of individuals with diabetes, significantly diminishing their life quality. The main aim of this research is to assess the impact of these two therapeutic approaches influence pain reduction and overall quality of life in this patient demographic. Given the higher incidence of periarthritis of shoulder among diabetic patients, the research underscores the necessity of tailoring treatment strategies to this group, as existing literature predominantly focuses on the broader population. The investigation seeks to discern the relative efficacy of Muscle Energy Technique (MET) and Kalternborn Mobilisation Technique in mitigating pain associated with shoulder Periarthritis in people with diabetes. Key metrics for assessing the interventions' success include the Numerical Pain Rating Scale and the Shoulder Pain and Disability Index. The research methodology entails enlisting diabetic subjects diagnosed with Periarthritis of the Shoulder, their subsequent random allocation into two distinct groups for treatment, and collecting and analysing data pre- and post-intervention to gauge the therapeutic impact. The study meticulously outlines its experimental design, participant recruitment and randomization processes, intervention protocols, and analytical methods to evaluate outcomes. Doing so aims to fill a critical gap in the current understanding of effective pain management strategies for diabetic patients suffering from Periarthritis of the Shoulder. The anticipated findings from this research are poised to significantly contribute to optimising care and management for this patient subset, potentially establishing a preferred treatment modality based on empirical evidence. This research article sheds light on the comparative effectiveness of two distinct physical therapy techniques in alleviating pain for diabetic individuals with Periarthritis of Shoulder arthritis. A rigorous experimental setup and systematic analysis aim to identify the most efficacious intervention, informing clinical practices and enhancing the quality of life for this patient population. The study's implications extend beyond immediate pain relief, aiming to provide a foundation for more personalized and effective treatment approaches for diabetic patients grappling with shoulder periarthritis.

Georgiannos et al., (2017) published that, adhensive capsulitis is marked by significant pain and limited range of motion, which profoundly impacts daily activities and quality of life. The underlying mechanisms of Adhesive Capsulitis of the Shoulder (ACS) remain elusive, which complicates its management. Clinically, Adhesive Capsulitis of the Shoulder manifests through progressive stages of pain and stiffness, and recovery is not always complete, with some individuals experiencing persistent limitations. The treatment regimen for Adhesive Capsulitis of the Shoulder is tiered based on the severity and duration of symptoms. Initially, conservative approaches are recommended, which include the use of anti-inflammatory drugs, steroid or hyaluronate injections, and dedicated physiotherapy sessions. These treatments aim to reduce inflammation and pain, gradually improving shoulder mobility. As the condition advances, or if initial treatments fail to provide relief, more invasive procedures may be considered. These include suprascapular nerve block, distension arthrography, and manipulation under anesthesia, which is geared towards more significant relief and is employed in the intermediate stages of the disease. For patients with severe and recalcitrant Adhesive Capsulitis of the Shoulder, surgical interventions such as arthroscopic capsular release or open surgical release may be necessary. These procedures aim to reduce the tightness by releasing the joint capsule, thereby improving the range of motion. Despite the variety of available treatments, there needs to be more consensus on the optimal management strategies for Adhesive Capsulitis of the Shoulder. This ambiguity largely stems from the reliance on clinical experience and observational studies rather than robust, evidence-based research. The literature on Adhesive Capsulitis of the Shoulder treatment predominantly includes case series and retrospective comparative studies, which do not provide the evidence necessary to formulate standardized treatment protocols. Consequently, medicines such as oral steroids and intra-articular injections, while beneficial in the short term, need to have well-established long-term efficacy. The review underscores a critical need for more rigorous research to develop evidence-based guidelines for Adhesive Capsulitis of the Shoulder management. Randomized controlled trials and larger cohort studies would be instrumental in clarifying the effectiveness of different treatment modalities and establishing a standardized approach to managing this debilitating condition. This review serves as a valuable resource for healthcare professionals, offering a comprehensive overview of the current understanding and treatment options for Adhesive Capsulitis of the Shoulder. It encourages clinicians to integrate the available evidence with their clinical expertise and patient preferences to tailor treatment plans that optimize outcomes for individuals suffering from this challenging condition. In summary, while managing Periarthritis of shoulder is multifaceted and continues to evolve, the current approach is characterized by a step-wise escalation of treatments from conservative to more invasive options based on the patient's response to therapy. The ongoing debate and the recognized need for further studies highlight the dynamic nature of Adhesive Capsulitis of the Shoulder and the pursuit of more definitive treatment strategies.

Kolathuru et al., (2023) stated that this study, provides a comprehensive overview of the causes, risk factors, stages, treatment options, recent advances, and future directives for managing this condition. Periarthritis of shoulder, is a condition that causes pain, stiffness, and limited range of motion in the shoulder joint. The authors divide the stages of periarthritis of shoulder into four distinct phases based on clinical presentation and arthroscopic appearance. Stage I is characterized by shoulder pain with preserved motion, while Stage II involves stiffness with early adhesion formation. Stage III is marked by a global loss of range of motion and significant adhesions, and Stage IV exhibits persistent stiffness with minimal pain and advanced adhesions. The article also explores the histological and MRI staging of periarthritis of shoulder, providing a deeper understanding of the condition's progression. Regarding treatment, the article discusses various conservative modalities, including non-steroidal anti-inflammatory drugs (NSAIDs), oral corticosteroids, intraarticular injections, suprascapular nerve block, physical therapy, and arthrographic joint distension. These options aim to reduce pain, improve range of motion, and prevent further adhesion formation. For refractory cases that do not respond to conservative treatment, surgical management options such as closed manipulation under anesthesia, arthroscopic capsular release, and open capsulotomy are considered. The article also highlights recent advances in treating periarthritis of shoulder, particularly platelet-rich plasma (PRP) and mesenchymal stromal cells (MSCs) for rotator cuff disorders. PRP has shown promising results in reducing histological grading without adverse effects, while MSCs and exosomes have demonstrated improved tendon healing and reduced re-tear rates. These innovative approaches offer potential new avenues for treating this challenging condition. Looking to the future, the authors discuss the potential of enzymatic capsulotomies using collagenase and Botox injections as emerging treatment options for periarthritis of shoulder. These novel approaches may provide less invasive alternatives to surgical interventions, potentially reducing recovery time and improving patient outcomes. In conclusion, the article emphasizes the importance of appropriate treatment modalities in decreasing morbidity and improving the functional quality of life for individuals with periarthritis of shoulder. By understanding the causes, risk factors, and stages of the condition, healthcare providers can develop personalized treatment plans that address each patient's unique needs. As research advances our understanding of periarthritis of shoulder, new and innovative treatment options may emerge, offering hope for those struggling with this debilitating condition.

As a conclusion, the studies above aim to assess pain reduction and quality of life improvements through a structured methodology, including random participant allocation and evaluation using the Numerical Pain Rating Scale and Shoulder Pain and Disability Index. The findings are expected to enhance treatment strategies for this demographic, addressing a significant gap in current literature and potentially establishing preferred therapeutic interventions based on empirical evidence.

1.12.2 Posterior Capsule Tightness

Yavanika (2023) conducted a study about the effectiveness of the Muscle Energy Technique (MET) and Cross Body Stretch was compared to determine their impact on alleviating posterior shoulder tightness and pain in patients suffering from various shoulder conditions. This study included a total of 68 participants who were experiencing shoulder pain due to issues such as rotator cuff problems, periarthritis of shoulder, and labral lesions. These participants were divided into two distinct groups for the trial. Group 1 was treated with MET in conjunction with conventional therapies, whereas Group 2 underwent Cross

Body Stretch along with the standard treatment protocols. The primary objective of this research was to explore the potential benefits of these techniques in mitigating posterior shoulder tightness, a prevalent condition that can significantly hinder shoulder mobility. To qualify for the study, participants were required to have experienced shoulder pain for a minimum duration of three months and exhibit a global restriction in the range of motion of the glenohumeral joint. To assess the outcomes, pain levels were quantitatively measured using the Numeric Pain Rating Scale (NPRS), and the degree of shoulder horizontal adduction was evaluated using a goniometer. The collected data was then analyzed using SPSS software, where normality tests were conducted to determine the data distribution. The results indicated no significant difference between the two groups regarding improvement in shoulder horizontal adduction and reduction in pain levels. This suggests that MET and Cross Body Stretch are equally effective when combined with conventional treatments to manage posterior shoulder tightness and associated pain. However, the study did have some limitations that should be considered when interpreting the results. One of the primary constraints was the relatively short duration of the intervention, which lasted only four weeks. Additionally, the study did not include follow-up assessments to evaluate the long-term effects of the treatments. Given these findings, the study proposes several recommendations for future research. It suggests that subsequent studies should consider including measurements of shoulder strength and examining the kinetics of the shoulder joint to gain a more comprehensive understanding of the effects of these treatments. Moreover, implementing longer-term interventions with follow-up evaluations could provide deeper insights into the sustained efficacy of MET and Cross Body Stretch in treating shoulder conditions. The trial was conducted with ethical oversight and received approval from the Max Healthcare Ethical Board, ensuring the study adhered to the necessary ethical standards in medical research. In conclusion, this study contributes valuable information to physical therapy by comparing the effectiveness of MET and Cross Body Stretch in treating posterior shoulder tightness and pain. While both techniques proved equally effective when used alongside conventional treatments, further research is needed to explore their long-term benefits and potential impacts on shoulder function and strength.

Winkelmann (2020) published that, handball is a physically demanding sport that involves repetitive overhead throwing motions, which can lead to adaptations in the shoulder joint and surrounding soft tissues. These adaptations may contribute to developing shoulder injuries, particularly in elite youth handball players exposed to high training loads. A recent study aimed to investigate the differences in posterior shoulder capsule thickness and glenohumeral rotation between the throwing and non-throwing shoulders of youth elite handball players. The study included 63 youth elite handball players (33 boys and 30 girls) with a mean age of 13.6 ± 0.9 years. The researchers assessed various shoulder parameters, including glenohumeral internal and external rotation range of motion, humeral retroversion, and posterior capsule thickness. Measurements were taken using a manual goniometer and a portable ultrasound device. The study calculated sports-specific differences between the throwing and non-throwing shoulders and correlations with posterior capsule thickness. The study found significant differences in internal rotation, external rotation, and humeral retroversion between elite youth handball players' throwing and non-throwing shoulders. The posterior capsule of the throwing shoulder was 1.21 times thicker (95% confidence interval: 1.1-1.3) than that of the non-throwing shoulder (1.3 ± 0.3 mm vs. 1.2 ± 0.2 mm, $P < .0001$). This difference was observed in both male and female players. However, the study found no correlations between posterior capsule thickness and sports-specific glenohumeral measurements in the throwing shoulder, such as internal rotation deficit, glenohumeral internal rotation deficit (GIRD), or humeral retroversion. The loss of internal rotation did not correlate with posterior capsule thickness. The findings of this study contribute to the understanding of adaptations in the shoulders of overhead-throwing athletes, particularly in youth elite handball players. The 21% difference in posterior capsule thickness between the throwing and non-throwing shoulders highlights the importance of identifying sport-specific adaptations in the glenohumeral joint. The lack of correlation between posterior capsule thickness and internal rotation deficits suggests that other soft-tissue factors may be responsible for developing posterior shoulder tightness and losing internal rotation in elite youth handball players. These factors could include changes in the rotator cuff muscles, capsular contracture, or muscular imbalances. The study emphasizes the importance of understanding soft-tissue adaptations in handball players to improve screening and injury prevention strategies. By identifying physiological adaptations and distinguishing them from pathologies, sports medicine professionals can develop targeted interventions to reduce the risk of overuse shoulder injuries in youth elite handball players. In conclusion, this study found significant differences in posterior capsule thickness between youth elite handball players' throwing and non-throwing shoulders. However, the increased thickness did not correlate with greater internal rotation deficits, suggesting that other soft-tissue factors may contribute to posterior shoulder tightness and loss of internal rotation in this population. The findings highlight the importance of investigating sport-specific adaptations in the glenohumeral joint to enhance screening, injury prevention, and return-to-competition strategies for elite youth handball players. Future research should focus on identifying the specific soft-tissue factors responsible for developing shoulder injuries in this population and developing targeted interventions to mitigate these risks.

Rabbani & BV (2021) stated that, this study aimed to evaluate the effectiveness of combining muscle energy technique with sleeper stretch in addressing posterior shoulder tightness among tennis players. Posterior shoulder tightness is a common issue linked to bony and soft tissue adaptations resulting from the repetitive rotational and distractive forces acting on the glenohumeral joint during overhead activities. These forces can lead to soft tissue microtrauma, shoulder lesions, and conditions such as shoulder impingement syndrome, labral lesions, and rotator cuff pathology. Lengthening the soft tissues in the posterior aspect of the shoulder is crucial for proper shoulder range of motion, kinematics, and kinetics. The study involved 50 tennis players who met the Gleno-humeral internal rotation deficit (GIRD) criteria, a condition characterized by limited shoulder joint internal rotation. The participants underwent a treatment regimen that combined muscle energy technique and sleeper stretch, performed three days per week for four weeks. The muscle energy technique involved protocols targeting the glenohumeral joint horizontal abductors and external rotators. The subjects performed the sleeper stretch under the guidance of a therapist. This stretch is designed to increase the shoulder's internal rotation and posterior capsule extensibility. The outcome measures included shoulder range of motion for adduction and internal rotation, assessed using a goniometer, and the Shoulder Pain and Disability Index (SPADI) to evaluate pain and disability levels. After the intervention, the results showed significant improvements in shoulder adduction, internal rotation, and SPADI scores. These findings indicate enhanced range of motion and reduced pain and disability in the shoulder joint among the tennis players who received the combined treatment. The study highlighted the importance of addressing posterior shoulder tightness in tennis players, as it can contribute to various shoulder pathologies and impair performance. The combination of muscle energy technique and sleeper stretch demonstrated promising results in increasing shoulder range of motion and reducing pain and disability associated with posterior shoulder tightness. The study suggested the need for further research to explore the long-term effects of this intervention and its applicability in various populations and performance levels. Additionally, investigating the individual contributions of muscle energy technique and sleeper stretch could provide valuable insights into the most effective treatment approach. The combination of muscle energy technique with sleeper stretch demonstrated potential benefits in managing shoulder issues related to repetitive overhead motions in sports like tennis. Addressing posterior shoulder tightness through these interventions may help prevent shoulder injuries, improve performance, and enhance overall shoulder health in tennis players.

Hall et al. (2020) published that this study, the research was designed to evaluate the inter-session reliability of three clinical tests commonly used to diagnose posterior shoulder tightness (PST) over 6 to 10 weeks. The tests assessed were Glenohumeral horizontal adduction (HorAdd), Shoulder internal rotation at 90-degree abduction (GHj-IR), and Low flexion (LF). The study successfully demonstrated good inter-session intra-rater reliability for all three tests, with Intraclass Correlation Coefficient (ICC) values ranging between 0.86 and 0.88. The standard error of measurement (SEM) was calculated for each test, revealing SEM values of 3.7° for HorAdd, 4.8° for GHj-IR, and 3.5° for LF. The minimum detectable change (MDC) was also determined, with HorAdd showing an MDC of 10.2°, GHj-IR 13.3°, and LF 9.7°. These metrics are crucial as they indicate the smallest statistically significant and detectable changes beyond measurement error. The criteria proposed for defining PST included a side-to-side difference of at least 10° in two clinical tests (GHj-IR, HorAdd, and LF) or a difference of 20° or more in any single test. This definition is based on the quantifiable and reliable measures obtained from the clinical tests. Previous literature primarily focused on the intra-session reliability of these tests, with reported ICC values ranging from 0.72 to 0.99 for GHj-IR, 0.91 to 0.94 for HorAdd, and 0.90 to 0.95 for LF. However, there was a notable gap in the literature regarding inter-session reliability data, which this study aimed to address by extending the testing period to between 6 and 10 weeks. The findings from this study underscore the robustness of the three PST measures in terms of inter-session reliability among asymptomatic participants. The high ICC values obtained suggest that the reliability of these tests is maintained over time, regardless of the presence of symptoms. This is significant as it supports the use of these tests in clinical and research settings to assess changes in shoulder tightness over time. In conclusion, this study fills a critical gap in the existing literature by providing valuable inter-session reliability data and contributes to the clinical understanding of PST. By establishing reliable and precise measurements, healthcare professionals can better diagnose and manage posterior shoulder tightness, ultimately enhancing patient care and treatment outcomes. The proposed definition of PST, grounded in empirical evidence, offers a clear and practical guideline for clinicians to follow in their practice.

The studies reviewed focus on various methods for treating and understanding posterior shoulder tightness, particularly in athletes. Yavanika (2023) compared Muscle Energy Technique (MET) and Cross Body Stretch, finding both equally effective in reducing shoulder tightness and pain when combined with conventional treatments. Winkelmann (2020) examined shoulder adaptations in youth handball players, noting increased posterior capsule thickness in the throwing shoulder, but no correlation with internal rotation deficits. Rabbani & BV (2021) assessed MET and sleeper stretch in tennis players, reporting improvements in shoulder range of motion and reduced pain. Hall et al. (2020) tested clinical methods for diagnosing posterior shoulder tightness, confirming the reliability of three tests. These studies emphasize the importance of targeted interventions in managing shoulder tightness in athletes.

1.12.3 Prevalence of Periarthritis Shoulder

Inayat et al., (2017) stated that, the study on frozen shoulder (FS) among the diabetic population in Pakistan unveiled some noteworthy findings that shed light on the prevalence and determinants of this debilitating condition. One of the most striking revelations was the significantly higher incidence of frozen shoulder among female patients, with the prevalence rate being 2.66 times greater compared to their male counterparts. This gender disparity highlights the need for heightened vigilance and targeted interventions for women with diabetes who may be at an elevated risk of developing frozen shoulder. Another key observation was the slightly higher frequency of frozen shoulder among patients on insulin therapy, either as a standalone treatment or in combination with oral anti-diabetic medications. This finding underscores the potential impact of insulin on the development of frozen shoulder, possibly due to the complex interplay between insulin, glucose metabolism, and inflammatory processes within the body. The study also revealed a concerning association between uncontrolled blood glucose levels over the past three months and an increased risk of developing shoulder pain, with a 1.5 times higher rate observed in patients with poor glycemic control. This finding reinforces the importance of maintaining optimal blood sugar levels, as persistent hyperglycemia may contribute to developing and exacerbating frozen shoulder various pathophysiological mechanisms. Interestingly, the study found that a positive family history of similar ailments was also linked to a 1.5 times higher rate of frozen shoulder development, suggesting a potential genetic or environmental component that warrants further investigation. However, factors such as age distribution, duration of diabetes, and regular exercise did not exhibit a significant relationship with the occurrence of frozen shoulder in this study population. The study's findings underscore the critical need for heightened awareness, early screening, and updated clinical knowledge among healthcare professionals to improve the diagnosis and management of frozen shoulder in diabetic populations. Implementing mass awareness campaigns, particularly targeting female patients with diabetes, could play a pivotal role in facilitating early detection and appropriate interventions. Furthermore, the study emphasizes the importance of glycemic control and early management of frozen shoulder in diabetic patients. Effective strategies for maintaining optimal blood sugar levels, coupled with timely interventions for frozen shoulder, could mitigate the risk of developing this debilitating condition and alleviate its associated symptoms. While the study provides valuable insights, further research is recommended to validate these findings and explore the association between frozen shoulder and diabetes in more extensive and diverse populations. Such research endeavours could unravel additional determinants, elucidate underlying mechanisms, and pave the way for tailored preventive and therapeutic approaches, ultimately improving the quality of life for diabetic patients at risk of frozen shoulder. In conclusion, the study on frozen shoulder in the Pakistani diabetic population has shed light on the significant burden of this condition, particularly among women, and the potential impact of factors such as insulin therapy, poor glycemic control, and family history. By addressing these findings through targeted interventions, awareness campaigns, and further research, the healthcare community can take strides towards mitigating the detrimental effects of frozen shoulder and improving the overall well-being of diabetic patients.

Cao et al. (2022) aimed to investigate the incidence of periarthritis of shoulder and identify risk factors for its onset in middle-aged and elderly subjects within one year of being discharged from a hospital where they received intravenous infusion. The researchers included 1,900 subjects in their study, dividing them into two equal groups based on the mean daily duration of intravenous infusion they received: 950 subjects received infusions for 2 hours or less per day, while the other 950 received infusions for 3 hours or more daily. The results showed that the overall cumulative incidence rate of periarthritis of shoulder within one year of hospital discharge was 5.2%. Interestingly, most cases of periarthritis of shoulder (66.3%) were diagnosed within the first 6 months after discharge. This finding suggests that the period immediately following hospitalization with intravenous infusion is a critical time for the development of periarthritis of shoulder in this population. The study identified several risk factors significantly associated with the onset of periarthritis of shoulder. These included a mean daily duration of intravenous infusion of 3 hours or more, a hospital stays lasting between 11 and 30 days, a body mass index (BMI) of 25 kg/m^2 or higher, being between 56 and 70 years old, and having diabetes. These factors independently increased the risk of developing a periarthritis of shoulder within one year of hospital discharge. Using multivariate logistic regression analysis, the researchers determined that subjects who received intravenous infusions for 3 hours or more per day had a higher risk of periarthritis of shoulder than those who received infusions for 2 hours or less daily. Additionally, subjects hospitalized for 11 to 30 days had a greater risk than those hospitalized for 10 days or less. Being overweight or obese (BMI $\geq$ 25 kg/m^2) in the 56 to 70-year-old age group or having diabetes also significantly increased the likelihood of developing periarthritis of shoulder. While this study provides valuable insights into the incidence and risk factors for periarthritis of shoulders in middle-aged and elderly individuals following hospitalization with intravenous infusion, it is important to acknowledge its limitations. The study analyzed subjects from a single centre with a relatively small sample size. Furthermore, the baseline characteristics between the exposure groups were not matched, potentially influencing the results. Despite these limitations, the study's findings have important implications for clinical practice. The authors conclude that middle-aged and elderly patients who receive intravenous infusion during hospitalization have a higher cumulative incidence rate of periarthritis of shoulder compared to the general population. By accurately identifying risk factors, healthcare providers can implement timely interventions, such as appropriate exercises, to help reduce the incidence of periarthritis of shoulders in this vulnerable population. In addition to the risk factors identified in the study by Cao et al., other research has shown that a periarthritis of shoulder can be effectively managed through a combination of conservative treatments. These may include oral medications like non-steroidal anti-inflammatory drugs (NSAIDs), physical therapy, exercise, steroid injections, and hydrodilatation. Treatment approaches may vary depending on the stage of periarthritis of shoulder, with pain management being a primary focus in the early stages and range of motion exercises becoming more important as the condition progresses. Specific exercises are particularly beneficial for individuals with periarthritis of shoulders. A study by Surrey Physio highlighted five top exercises, including the football supporter shoulder exercise, rocking the baby shoulder exercise, and wall crawl. These exercises aim to improve shoulder mobility and reduce pain and stiffness associated with a periarthritis of shoulder. Moreover, Sharma et al.'s randomized controlled trial investigated the effects of neuromuscular exercises compared to strengthening exercises on pain and active range of motion in individuals with idiopathic periarthritis of shoulders. The study found that when combined with regular physical therapy, neuromuscular exercises significantly improved pain scores and active range of motion in shoulder flexion, internal rotation, and external rotation compared to strengthening exercises. In conclusion, the study by Cao et al. provides valuable insights into the incidence and risk factors for periarthritis of shoulders in middle-aged and elderly individuals following hospitalization with intravenous infusion. By identifying characteristics such as longer duration of intravenous infusion, prolonged hospital stays, higher BMI, older age, and diabetes, healthcare providers can implement targeted interventions to reduce the risk of periarthritis of shoulder in this population. Additionally, a comprehensive approach to treatment, including medications, physical therapy, and specific exercises, can effectively manage periarthritis of shoulder and improve patient outcomes. Further research is needed to validate these findings and explore optimal prevention and treatment strategies for periarthritis of shoulders in various patient populations. The systematic review of the global prevalence and incidence of shoulder pain highlighted several crucial aspects that should be considered when interpreting and applying the findings. Firstly, the reported prevalence rates exhibited substantial variations attributed to differences in the study populations. For instance, studies conducted in Mexico and Iran yielded contrasting results, underscoring the influence of factors such as age, occupation, co-morbid health conditions, and access to healthcare on an individual's likelihood of reporting musculoskeletal pain.

Lucas et al., (2022) reveals notable discrepancies in the reported prevalence and incidence rates of shoulder pain, primarily stemming from variations in study populations and methodologies. For example, despite employing similar methods, two studies conducted in Mexico as part of the COPCORD project yielded prevalence rates of 5.28% and 15.2%. This difference can be attributed to their distinct recruitment strategies, targeting urban versus rural populations. A similar trend of variability was observed in research from Iran. The review underscores the importance of factors such as age, occupation, and health literacy, which were not thoroughly examined and may impact the reporting of musculoskeletal pain. Interestingly, while the prevalence of shoulder pathology tends to rise with age, the reporting of pain decreases after age 65. This decline may be influenced by various lifestyle factors that warrant further investigation. One of the strengths of this review is its extensive search strategy, which incorporated a larger number of studies than previous reviews, particularly from a wide range of geographical locations. However, the review also has limitations, including the possibility of missing relevant studies due to its narrow search criteria and the exclusion of non-English research, which could lead to bias in the findings. Additionally, the authors pointed out that the heterogeneity of the included studies prevented them from performing a meta-analysis. Most of the studies reviewed exhibited a low risk of bias; however, common limitations were identified, such as the presence of non-representative target populations and inconsistent case definitions. The authors emphasize the need for standardized methodologies in future research endeavours to enhance the comparability and interpretation of epidemiological data related to shoulder pain. They urge healthcare professionals and policymakers to consider these variations when assessing prevalence and incidence rates from individual studies. In summary, Lucas et al.'s review highlights the complexities surrounding the epidemiology of shoulder pain, calling attention to the factors influencing variability in reported rates. The findings advocate for improved research practices that could provide more reliable data and better-informed healthcare decisions.

Jacob et al., (2023) stated that, the research project was designed to explore the occurrence and contributing factors of periarthritis of shoulder among the elderly population in Germany. This condition, commonly known as frozen shoulder, is characterized by stiffness and pain in the shoulder joint. To achieve a comprehensive understanding, the study drew on data from the Disease Analyzer database, focusing on two groups of older adults. The first group examined was those aged 65 years and older in 2021, with the aim of determining the prevalence of periarthritis of shoulder within this demographic. The second group consisted of older adults who had been diagnosed with periarthritis of shoulder between 2010 and 2021. This segment of the study was particularly focused on identifying physical and psychiatric conditions that might be linked to the development of the disorder in these patients. The study's findings were quite revealing. In 2021, the one-year prevalence of periarthritis of shoulder in older people was 0.4%, while the lifetime prevalence was significantly higher at 2.4%. These statistics underscore that while the condition may not be extremely common within a single year, a considerable number of older adults are likely to experience it at some point in their lives. Moreover, the research identified 12 conditions significantly associated with periarthritis of shoulder development. Among these, the conditions with the most substantial impact were other and unspecified osteoarthritis, injuries to the shoulder and upper arm, and injuries to the thorax. These findings suggest that physical trauma or underlying joint disorders could play a critical role in the onset of periarthritis of shoulder in older adults. The study illuminates the prevalence and associated risk factors of periarthritis of shoulder in older adults and emphasizes the complexity of this medical condition. It highlights the need for healthcare providers to be aware of the various factors that could predispose someone to develop this painful and debilitating condition. Understanding these risk factors is crucial for early diagnosis and effective disease management. Furthermore, the research underscores the importance of ongoing investigation into the epidemiology of periarthritis of shoulder. With an aging global population, the prevalence of such conditions is likely to increase, making it imperative for medical research to continue exploring the mechanisms and risk factors associated with these diseases and effective strategies for prevention and treatment. In conclusion, this study provides valuable insights into the prevalence and risk factors of periarthritis of shoulder among older adults in Germany. By utilizing a robust database and focusing on a specific age group, the researchers have contributed significantly to the understanding of this condition. The findings highlight the need for further research to explore the underlying causes and potential treatments for periarthritis of shoulder, aiming to improve the quality of life for the aging population who may be affected by this condition. This research is a step forward in geriatric medicine and opens new scientific exploration and clinical practice avenues.

Several studies have explored the prevalence and risk factors of frozen shoulder (FS) and periarthritis of the shoulder, highlighting important patterns and contributing factors. These studies collectively highlight the complexity of shoulder conditions, emphasizing the importance of early diagnosis, risk factor identification, and targeted treatment strategies, especially in vulnerable populations like women, the elderly, and diabetics.

1.12.4 Sign and Symptoms

Brindisino et al., (2022) published that, it has been observed that patients suffering from Frozen Shoulder Contracture Syndrome who also report symptoms of anxiety and depression tend to perceive greater pain, exhibit lower functional capabilities, and experience a diminished quality of life. The review, however, leaves open the question of whether these psychological symptoms precede the onset of Frozen Shoulder Contracture Syndrome or are a consequence of dealing with the condition. The concept of a unique "periarthritis of shoulder personality" that predisposes individuals to Frozen Shoulder Contracture Syndrome was explored, but the findings were inconsistent. The review suggests that the inherent characteristics of Frozen Shoulder Contracture Syndrome, such as the way it manifests and its effects on pain and disability, particularly in middle-aged working adults, might play a role in the emergence of psychological issues. The presence of anxiety and depression among individuals with Frozen Shoulder Contracture Syndrome is strongly linked to sleep disturbances. These sleep issues contribute to increased physical and psychological exhaustion, further impairing the patient's quality of life. The interrelation between sleep disturbances and psychological health is highlighted as a significant concern for individuals with Frozen Shoulder Contracture Syndrome The review points out that delays in obtaining an accurate diagnosis of Frozen Shoulder Contracture Syndrome can exacerbate psychological distress, such as anxiety and depression. The prolonged uncertainty about prognosis and the escalation of pain-related disability during the wait for diagnosis can severely impact the psychological well-being of patients. Educating patients about pain neuroscience has proven beneficial in managing musculoskeletal pain, including Frozen Shoulder Contracture Syndrome. Such educational interventions can aid patients in reconceptualizing their pain and enhancing their coping strategies, thereby reducing pain, improving function, and decreasing disability. For effective management of Frozen Shoulder Contracture Syndrome healthcare providers must assess patients' psychological aspects. Recognizing the predictive value of these psychological factors can inform the integration of therapeutic strategies that address both the physical and psychological dimensions of the condition. The review advocates for further research into additional psychological factors such as expectations, fear, and optimism better to understand their impact on the prognosis of Frozen Shoulder Contracture Syndrome (FSCS). Future studies should aim to identify individuals at higher risk and assess the effectiveness of treatments that incorporate a psychosocial perspective. This systematic review underscores the critical need to consider psychological factors in both the assessment and treatment of FSCS. By addressing these aspects, healthcare professionals can enhance therapeutic outcomes and improve the overall well-being of patients suffering from this debilitating condition.

Ramirez J (2019) stated that, periarthritis of shoulder, is characterized by progressive shoulder pain and restricted range of motion, particularly in external rotation. While the underlying cause is often idiopathic, it is more prevalent among individuals with diabetes mellitus and hypothyroidism. The diagnosis of periarthritis of shoulder is primarily clinical, based on the patient's history and physical examination findings. Imaging modalities, such as non-contrast magnetic resonance imaging (MRI), can confirm the diagnosis and rule out other potential shoulder pathologies. Specific MRI findings, such as thickening of the coracohumeral ligament, rotator interval infiltration, and axillary recess thickening, have been shown to have high specificity for periarthritis of shoulder. Traditionally, periarthritis of shoulder was believed to follow a self-limiting course, progressing through three distinct phases: the painful freezing stage, the stiffening frozen stage, and the thawing recovery stage. The condition was thought to resolve spontaneously within one to two years without treatment. However, recent clinical evidence challenges this notion, suggesting that untreated periarthritis of shoulder may result in persistent functional limitations and long-term disability. The optimal treatment approach for periarthritis of shoulder remains uncertain, with various nonsurgical and surgical options available. Nonsurgical treatments include nonsteroidal anti-inflammatory drugs (NSAIDs) for pain relief, corticosteroid injections, physiotherapy, acupuncture, and hydro dilatation (distension of the joint capsule with fluid). Combining physiotherapy and corticosteroid injections may improve symptoms compared to physiotherapy alone. Additionally, the combination of hydro dilatation and corticosteroid injection may expedite the recovery of a pain-free range of motion. In cases where nonsurgical treatments fail to provide significant improvement, surgical interventions may be considered. These include manipulation under anaesthesia, where the shoulder is forcibly moved through its range of motion while the patient is under general anaesthesia, and arthroscopic capsular release, which involves surgically releasing the contracted joint capsule. It is essential to consider alternative diagnoses when evaluating shoulder pain, as other conditions, such as rotator cuff pathology, glenohumeral osteoarthritis, and shoulder instability, can present with similar symptoms. Diagnostic testing, including blood tests and imaging studies (e.g., X-rays, MRI), may be necessary to rule out other potential pathologies. While managing periarthritis of shoulder remains a challenge, physiotherapy, corticosteroid injections, and hydro dilatation have shown promising results in improving the range of motion and reducing pain. Early intervention and a multidisciplinary approach involving physiotherapists, orthopaedic surgeons, and other healthcare professionals may improve outcomes. In cases of persistent symptoms despite nonsurgical treatments, referral to an orthopaedic surgeon for consideration of surgical interventions may be warranted.

As a conclusion, the review calls for more research into the psychological factors that affect FSCS, advocating for an integrated approach that addresses both physical and mental health aspects to improve patient outcomes. Moreover, early intervention and a multidisciplinary approach are essential for better outcomes, with alternative diagnoses being considered in the differential diagnosis of shoulder pain.

1.12.5 Effect of Grade 3 Maitland Joint Mobilization

Zavala-González et al., (2018) stated that, the table provided offers a comprehensive overview of research studies on applying mobilization techniques for treating shoulder disorders, particularly periarthritis of shoulder. These studies explore a variety of interventions, outcomes, and comparisons, emphasizing the impact on pain alleviation, enhancement of range of motion (ROM), functionality, and reduction of disability in affected patients. The research primarily investigates the comparative effectiveness of different mobilization strategies, such as the Kaltenborn and Maitland techniques. It delves into the specifics of applying anterior versus posterior glide mobilization and the distinctions between high-grade and low-grade mobilization methods. The collective findings from these studies are instrumental in shedding light on the efficacy of various mobilization techniques in managing shoulder conditions. By comparing methodologies like the Kaltenborn and Maitland techniques and different mobilization approaches (anterior vs. posterior glide), the research helps delineate which methods might be more beneficial in specific therapeutic contexts. This is particularly relevant for clinicians and therapists seeking to optimize treatment strategies for patients suffering from periarthritis of shoulder. Moreover, these studies underscore the significance of integrating mobilization techniques into comprehensive treatment plans to enhance shoulder function and mitigate pain in patients with periarthritis of shoulder. The insights gained from these investigations contribute to a better understanding of effective therapeutic interventions and guide clinical practices in managing periarthritis of shoulder syndrome and other related shoulder impairments. The research encapsulated in the table provides a critical evaluation of mobilization techniques, offering evidence-based guidance on the most effective strategies for improving patient outcomes in periarthritis of shoulder. Through systematic reviews and randomized controlled trials, the studies assess the impact of various mobilization methods on pain, ROM, functionality, and disability, thereby informing and refining therapeutic approaches for managing complex shoulder conditions.

Lee et al., (2023) stated that, this study aimed to systematically investigate the effects of exercise interventions, both alone and combined with joint mobilization techniques, on patients suffering from Adhesive capsulitis (AC) or periarthritis of shoulder. Adhesive capsulitis is a debilitating condition characterized by severe shoulder pain and significant restriction in active and passive range of motion (ROM). This systematic review and meta-analysis synthesized evidence from nine peer-reviewed studies published between 2000 and 2021 that met specific inclusion criteria for Adhesive capsulitis, exercise, and joint mobilization interventions. The analysis revealed that exercise alone and combined with joint mobilization demonstrated large effect sizes in improving shoulder ROM and subjective outcomes like pain and function for Adhesive capsulitis patients. However, combining the two interventions showed statistically significant superiority over exercise alone in enhancing specific ROM measures. Patients who performed exercises integrated with joint mobilization techniques experienced greater improvements in shoulder flexion, extension, internal rotation, external rotation, and abduction ROM than those who only did exercises. On the other hand, patients who underwent exercise interventions without joint mobilization exhibited higher effect sizes for improvement in subjective function, as measured by tools like the Shoulder Pain and Disability Index (SPADI) and pain relief. This finding suggests that while joint mobilization augments ROM recovery when combined with exercise, exercise alone may substantially alleviate pain and improve self-reported functional ability in Adhesive capsulitis patients. The study underscored the significant effectiveness of exercise interventions in treating Adhesive capsulitis, particularly for pain management. Exercises can be easily incorporated into daily life routines, making them a preferable first-line treatment option. The authors recommended preferentially prescribing exercise programs for Adhesive capsulitis patients, with the addition of joint mobilization techniques when enhanced ROM recovery is desired. Furthermore, the study discussed the potential benefits of incorporating virtual reality (VR) training and coracohumeral ligament stretching exercises into Adhesive capsulitis programs. VR-based interventions may enhance patient engagement and interest, while coracohumeral ligament stretches could specifically target ROM limitations caused by tightness in this anatomical structure. The authors emphasized tailoring exercise programs to individual patient needs, symptoms, and ROM deficits. By carefully assessing each patient's condition and adjusting the balance between exercise and joint mobilization components, rehabilitation programs can be optimized for maximum effectiveness. In conclusion, this systematic review and meta-analysis provided robust evidence supporting the significant positive effects of exercise interventions, both alone and combined with joint mobilization, on shoulder ROM, pain relief, and subjective function improvement in patients with periarthritis of shoulder. The authors recommended constructing rehabilitation exercise programs based on individual symptoms and adjusting the balance of exercise and joint mobilization to achieve optimal outcomes.

As a summary, these studies explored different mobilization methods, such as the Kaltenborn and Maitland techniques, and examined the impact of anterior versus posterior glide mobilization, as well as high-grade and low-grade approaches. These findings guide clinicians in choosing the most effective strategies for treating periarthritis of the shoulder. Additionally, the study emphasized the benefits of exercise as a first-line treatment, with the addition of joint mobilization when ROM recovery is prioritized. The authors also suggested incorporating innovative interventions like virtual reality training and targeted ligament stretching to further enhance rehabilitation outcomes, urging tailored exercise programs based on individual patient needs.

1.12.6 Effect of Modified Posterior Capsular Stretching

Gharisia et al. (2021) conducted a study to evaluated the effectiveness of a newly developed stretching technique called "Passive Glenohumeral Internal Rotation with Clam Shell Bridging" compared to the traditional modified sleeper stretch. The aim was to determine which approach was more beneficial for improving the internal rotation range of motion and reducing pain levels in overhead athletes suffering from glenohumeral internal rotation deficits (GIRD). The study involved 42 overhead athletes diagnosed with GIRD, with an average age of around 26, comprising 20 males and 22 females. The participants were randomly allocated to one of two intervention groups the novel stretching group or the traditional modified sleeper stretching group. Objective measurements were taken at three-time points: baseline, immediately after the intervention, and again at 4 weeks post-intervention. The primary outcome measure was the glenohumeral internal rotation range of motion (GHIR_ROM), assessed using a digital inclinometer. Self-reported pain levels were also evaluated using the Numeric Pain Rating Scale. The researchers ensured strict adherence to the study protocol, with 100% compliance reported in both groups. Additionally, the participants' baseline characteristics were comparable across the two groups. The results revealed that both stretching techniques led to statistically significant improvements in GHIR_ROM immediately after the intervention and at the 4-week follow-up compared to baseline measurements. Interestingly, the novel stretching group demonstrated slightly superior outcomes regarding increased internal rotation range of motion, although the difference between the two groups was not statistically significant. A notable distinction emerged when examining the effects on self-reported pain intensity. While the novel stretching group experienced a substantial and statistically significant reduction in pain levels over the 4 weeks, the traditional modified sleeper stretch group did not exhibit any substantial changes in pain scores. This finding suggests that the newly developed stretching technique more effectively alleviates shoulder pain in overhead athletes with GIRD. The authors highlighted that their findings align with previous research demonstrating the efficacy of stretching interventions for improving range of motion deficits in the shoulder joint. However, they acknowledged the need for further investigation into the long-term effects of the novel stretching technique and comparative studies with other commonly used stretching methods. In summary, the study by Gharisia et al. (2021) introduced a novel stretching approach called "Passive Glenohumeral Internal Rotation with Clam Shell Bridging" and compared its effectiveness to the traditional modified sleeper stretch in a population of overhead athletes with GIRD. Both techniques were similarly effective in enhancing the internal rotation range of motion. Still, the novel stretching method significantly reduced shoulder pain levels over 4 weeks. These findings suggest that the newly developed stretching technique may be a more appropriate choice for symptomatic overhead athletes seeking to alleviate pain while improving their shoulder mobility.

Tahran and Yeşilyaprak (2020) conducted research that focused on assessing the impact of altered posterior shoulder stretching exercises (PSSEs) on individuals suffering from subacromial impingement syndrome (SIS) and discrepancies in shoulder internal rotation. The study categorized participants into three groups: a modified cross-body stretch (MCS) group, a modified sleeper stretch (MSS) group, and a control group that did not receive the stretching interventions. The findings revealed enhancements across all groups regarding pain reduction, increased shoulder mobility, improved function, and decreased disability. Notably, the groups subjected to the stretching interventions exhibited superior outcomes in activity-related pain alleviation, internal rotation range of motion (ROM), functional capabilities, and disability levels compared to the control group. Despite these improvements, the study found no significant outcome differences between the MCS and MSS groups. The analysis further detailed that the MCS and MSS groups experienced notable advancements in reducing pain during activities, enhancing internal rotation ROM, and improving QuickDASH (Disabilities of the Arm, Shoulder, and Hand) scores, in stark contrast to the control group. Subsequent post hoc analysis underscored significant distinctions in internal rotation ROM improvements between the stretching and control groups, indicating that both stretching exercises contributed to clinically meaningful enhancements in QuickDASH scores. The research underscored the critical role of precise exercise prescription and the necessity of scapular stabilization in optimizing the efficacy of PSSEs. Moreover, the investigation illuminated the advantages of modified PSSEs for individuals afflicted with SIS and glenohumeral internal rotation deficit (GIRD). Incorporating these stretching exercises into the therapeutic regimen markedly improved outcomes related to pain during activities, internal rotation ROM, functionality, and disability, surpassing the results of treatment plans that excluded PSSEs. The study posited that modified PSSEs could be pivotal in diminishing subacromial pressure, thereby mitigating pain and enhancing functional capabilities in patients with SIS. In sum, the research by Tahran and Yeşilyaprak substantiates the efficacy of modified PSSEs in ameliorating pain, augmenting shoulder mobility, and enhancing both function and disability in individuals with SIS. The findings advocate for integrating stretching exercises into therapeutic programs to achieve significant improvements in various indicators of shoulder health and functionality. This study highlights the therapeutic potential of modified PSSEs and emphasizes the importance of tailored exercise interventions and scapular stabilization techniques in maximizing patient outcomes. Through its comprehensive analysis, the research contributes valuable insights into the management of SIS, offering a promising approach to improving the quality of life for those affected by this condition.

Keramat and Babur (2020) stated that, three primary stretches are commonly utilized to loosen the posterior capsule of the shoulder effectively: the cross-body stretch, the sleeper's stretch, and modified stretches. Research has demonstrated that both the cross-body stretch and the sleeper's stretch can enhance the range of internal rotation (IR) and external rotation (ER) in healthy individuals. However, these stretches do not adequately stabilize the scapula during the exercises. Consequently, a modified stretch has been developed and reported to achieve better outcomes in terms of IR and ER. Despite the benefits of these stretches, they fail to address the torsional stress on the posterior capsule, which is crucial for performing functional movements such as reaching up behind the back (RUBTB) and down behind the neck (RDBTN). The posterior capsule tightness is a significant factor in shoulder pathology, including scapular dyskinesis and glenohumeral rotation deficits, often linked to shoulder pain. The posterior capsule tends to become tight due to repetitive overload, particularly during the deceleration phase of throwing motions. This tightness can lead to hypertrophy of the posterior capsule, causing the humerus's greater tuberosity to translate superiorly, a common mechanism for subacromial impingement. Therefore, maintaining a lax posterior capsule is essential for optimal shoulder function. The cross-body stretch involves moving the arm across the body to stretch the posterior shoulder muscles and capsule. The sleeper's stretch is performed by lying on one side with the shoulder and elbow at 90 degrees of flexion, then using the opposite hand to apply a passive internal rotation force. Although these stretches increase IR and ER, they do not stabilize the scapula, which can lead to less effective results. A modified stretch has been introduced to address this issue, providing better stabilization of the scapula and improved outcomes in IR and ER. This modified stretch is designed to minimize symptoms of pain that can occur with the shoulder in a 90-degree flexed position. The modified sleeper stretch, for instance, is performed with the trunk rotated to minimize discomfort and enhance the stretch's effectiveness. However, all three stretches—cross-body, sleepers, and modified—do not sufficiently address the torsional stress required for RUBTB and RDBTN movements. Torsional stress on the posterior capsule is necessary for these functional movements, which involve complex shoulder mechanics and require high flexibility and stability. A pragmatic posterior capsular stretch (PPCS) has been developed to address this gap. The PPCS targets the posterior capsule in torsion to improve shoulder range of motion (ROM) and functional movements. Preliminary studies have shown that a single session of PPCS can significantly increase shoulder ROM in healthy subjects, bringing the ROM close to normal values. Despite these promising results, the current research on PPCS has limitations, including the need for a control group and the inability to generalize the findings. Future studies should involve multiple treatment sessions and include healthy subjects and individuals with shoulder pathology to validate PPCS's effectiveness further. In conclusion, while traditional stretches like the cross-body and sleeper's stretches can improve IR and ER, they do not stabilize the scapula or address the necessary torsional stress on the posterior capsule. The modified stretches offer better scapular stabilization but fail to address torsional stress. The PPCS presents a novel approach that could effectively improve shoulder ROM and functional movements, making it a valuable technique for preventing and rehabilitating shoulder pathologies, especially in overhead athletes. Further research is needed to confirm these findings and establish PPCS as a standard practice in shoulder rehabilitation.

As a conclusion, they emphasized the need for a modified stretch to address this issue and introduced a new posterior capsular stretch (PPCS) that targets torsional stress on the posterior capsule, improving shoulder range of motion and functional movements. Although the PPCS showed promising results, further research is needed to validate its effectiveness for shoulder rehabilitation. Together, these studies highlight the importance of targeted stretching techniques in managing shoulder conditions and suggest that novel approaches may offer enhanced outcomes in pain relief and range of motion for patients, particularly athletes.

1.12.17 Effect of Hotpack

Bin et al. (2021) stated that, the systematic review protocol on thermotherapy for shoulder pain is designed to rigorously evaluate the effectiveness and safety of thermotherapy as a treatment modality for this prevalent musculoskeletal condition. Shoulder pain significantly impacts a large segment of the population, prompting the need for effective treatment strategies. Thermotherapy, which involves the application of heat to affected areas, is a widely utilized approach. Despite its everyday use, there has been a need for rigorous scientific evaluation to determine its efficacy and safety for shoulder pain precisely. This systematic review aims to fill this gap by meticulously assessing the efficacy and safety of thermotherapy in treating shoulder pain. The review will involve a comprehensive search of several databases to identify randomized controlled trials (RCTs) that have investigated the effects of thermotherapy on shoulder pain. The review will adhere to stringent methodological standards to ensure the reliability and validity of the findings. The study selection criteria will be clearly defined to include only those RCTs that provide relevant data on the outcomes of interest. The search strategy will be meticulously planned to encompass relevant databases and include appropriate keywords and filters to capture all pertinent studies. Data collection will be systematically conducted, with two independent reviewers extracting data using a standardized form to minimize errors and bias. The assessment of the risk of bias in the included studies will be an integral part of the review, utilizing tools recommended by the Cochrane Collaboration. The treatment effects will be quantified, and meta-analytical techniques may be employed to synthesize data across studies, depending on the homogeneity of the studies' designs and outcomes. The review will follow the PRISMA-P guidelines and the Cochrane Handbook for Systematic Reviews of Interventions to guide its methodology. This adherence to internationally recognized standards will enhance the robustness and credibility of the review process. Additionally, the quality of evidence will be evaluated using the GRADE (Grading of Recommendations Assessment, Development, and Evaluation) system, which will facilitate clear and transparent recommendations based on the review findings. In summary, this systematic review will comprehensively evaluate the evidence regarding using thermotherapy for shoulder pain. By systematically assessing the effectiveness and safety of this treatment approach, the review aims to offer valuable insights that could inform clinical practices and guide future research in the management of shoulder pain. The findings could lead to improved treatment protocols that enhance patient outcomes in individuals suffering from this debilitating condition.

Raja et al., (2021) stated that the periarthritis of shoulder, is a debilitating condition characterized by progressive loss of shoulder joint mobility. It affects a significant portion of the population, particularly those with diabetes. A recent study compared the effectiveness of two mobilization techniques combined with hot pack therapy in improving shoulder abduction range in patients with periarthritis of shoulder. The study involved 80 subjects divided into two groups. Group A received anteroposterior glide mobilization, while Group B received caudal glide mobilization in combination with hot pack therapy. The researchers evaluated pain using the Visual Analogue Scale (VAS), shoulder range of motion (ROM) using a goniometer, and disability using the Shoulder Pain and Disability Index (SPADI). After a three-week protocol, both groups showed significant improvements in VAS scores, shoulder abduction ROM, and SPADI scores. However, Group B (caudal glide mobilization) demonstrated more substantial improvements than Group A (anteroposterior glide mobilization). The study concluded that caudal glide mobilization was more effective in reducing pain, increasing abduction ROM, and improving the SPADI index in patients with periarthritis of shoulder. The findings highlight the importance of proper mobilization techniques and hot pack therapy in managing periarthritis of shoulder. The researchers emphasized the need for further studies with larger sample sizes, longer durations, and control groups to enhance the accuracy of the results. Additionally, they noted the limitation of not implementing a strengthening program post-mobilization session and suggested its inclusion for better patient outcomes. The study provides valuable insights for clinicians and researchers in shoulder rehabilitation. Healthcare professionals can make informed decisions when treating patients with periarthritis of shoulder by understanding the effectiveness of different mobilization techniques. The results also pave the way for future research to explore the long-term effects of these interventions and their impact on patient quality of life. In conclusion, the study supports the effectiveness of caudal glide mobilization combined with hot pack therapy in improving shoulder abduction range in patients with capsulitis. However, further research is needed to validate these findings and explore additional treatment strategies for this challenging condition. By working collaboratively, healthcare professionals and researchers can continue to advance the understanding and management of periarthritis of shoulder, ultimately improving the quality of life for those affected by this debilitating. The study aimed to compare the therapeutic effects of moist hot packs combined with laser or ultrasound therapy in treating grade 1 and 2 rotator cuff injuries. The research involved 30 male subjects divided into two groups: group A received ultrasound therapy, and group B received laser therapy. Both groups were treated for 5 days a week over 4 weeks.

As a summary, these studies aim to assess randomized controlled trials (RCTs) investigating heat application for shoulder pain, adhering to rigorous methodological standards and using tools like GRADE for evidence evaluation. Moreover, the study called for further research to validate these findings and explore additional treatment strategies, including strengthening programs post-mobilization. Both studies contribute valuable insights into treatment protocols for shoulder pain and rehabilitation.

1.12.8 Effect of Visual Analgoue scale

Shirahama et al., (2021) stated that, understanding how people perceive and respond to conversational robots is crucial in human-robot interaction. A recent study delved into this intriguing domain by conducting a subjective evaluation experiment to assess the impressions formed during conversations with a talking robot. The researchers employed a powerful tool called the Visual Analog Scale (VAS) to capture the participants' intricate emotions and perceptions. The VAS is a psychometric scale that allows individuals to rate their subjective experiences along a continuous line rather than being confined to discrete categories. This approach offers a more nuanced and granular understanding of the participants' impressions, enabling researchers to capture the subtleties and gradations of their emotional responses. One key objective of the study was to identify patterns and similarities in the questions related to the robot's performance and the impressions formed during the conversations. To achieve this, the researchers employed a sophisticated statistical technique known as hierarchical cluster analysis. Hierarchical cluster analysis is a powerful tool that groups similar data points based on their characteristics, forming clusters that reveal underlying patterns and relationships. By applying this technique to the questions and responses from the subjective evaluation, the researchers could identify clusters of questions that elicited similar impressions and emotional responses from the participants. The analysis revealed a striking contrast between smooth and non-smooth conversations. Participants reported higher positive emotions, such as happiness and joy, in smooth discussions where the interaction flowed naturally and seamlessly. Conversely, in non-smooth conversations, where miscommunications or technical glitches hindered the interaction, participants experienced heightened negative emotions like sadness and anger. The researchers employed various statistical hypothesis-testing techniques to validate further and quantify their findings. One such technique was the Shapiro-Wilk test, which assesses whether a dataset follows a normal distribution—a crucial assumption for many parametric statistical tests. Additionally, the researchers conducted paired t-tests, a powerful statistical tool that compares the means of two related samples. In this case, the paired t-tests were used to compare the measurements obtained from smooth and non-smooth conversations, allowing the researchers to determine whether significant differences existed between the two conditions. Interestingly, the results of these statistical analyses indicated that the measurements for smooth conversations were not significantly greater than those for non-smooth conversations. This finding highlights the complexity and nuances involved in human-robot interactions, suggesting that factors beyond the mere smoothness of the conversation may influence people's impressions and emotional responses. One of the key strengths of the study lies in its use of the Visual Analog Scale (VAS) over traditional Likert scales. Likert scales, commonly used in surveys and questionnaires typically present participants with discrete response options (e.g., strongly agree, agree, neutral, disagree, strongly disagree). While widely used Likert scales have merits, they can sometimes fail to capture the subtleties and gradations of subjective experiences. Conversely, the VAS allows participants to express their impressions and emotions along a continuous line, providing a more nuanced and granular representation of their subjective experiences. This approach can be particularly valuable in human-robot interactions, where subtle cues and nuances can significantly impact people's perceptions and emotional responses. Furthermore, the study emphasized the importance of careful question design and hierarchical clustering in subjective evaluations. By thoughtfully crafting the questions and employing hierarchical cluster analysis, researchers can gain deeper insights into the underlying patterns and relationships within the data, ultimately enhancing their understanding of the complex dynamics in human-robot interactions. In conclusion, this study showcased the power of subjective evaluation techniques, such as the Visual Analog Scale and hierarchical cluster analysis, in unravelling the intricate impressions and emotional responses that arise during conversations with talking robots. By combining rigorous statistical analyses with careful question design and data exploration, researchers can unlock valuable insights that will shape the future of human-robot interactions, paving the way for more natural, engaging, and emotionally resonant experiences.

Shirahama et al., (2019) conducted a research paper presented at the 9th IIAE International Conference on Intelligent Systems and Image Processing 2022 delved into a comparative analysis of student reactions from Singapore and Japan to movie trailers, specifically focusing on the Arcane trailer showcased on YouTube. The core of the study involved a succinct questionnaire comprising five distinct questions (labelled Q1 through Q5), each designed with unique attributes and varying scales for response measurement. The participant pool consisted of 64 students from Singapore and 71 from Japan. Exploratory Data Analysis (EDA) was used to scrutinize the gathered data. This robust statistical approach facilitated a deep dive into the dataset through various graphical representations such as correlation coefficient visualizations, boxplots, histograms, and scatter plots. This comprehensive analysis shed light on the differing levels of engagement and emotional responses between the two groups, with Singaporean students displaying notably higher interest and emotional connectivity to the Arcane trailer than their Japanese counterparts. Further, the study employed hierarchical clustering techniques to segment the students into clusters based on their reactions to the trailer. This clustering reinforced the initial findings—highlighting the stronger and more positive reception among Singaporean students—and provided a nuanced understanding of the varied audience perceptions. An important aspect of the study was the implementation of the Visual Analog Scale (VAS) for data collection and analysis. The use of VAS was pivotal in quantifying the subtle nuances in student responses, thereby enhancing the precision of the analysis. The research also discussed the potential integration of the Likert Scale (LS) in future studies, especially in larger datasets, to compare its efficacy against the VAS. The researchers developed a predictive model utilizing linear regression techniques in an innovative stride. This model was designed to forecast the likelihood of students' interest in watching the full movie based on their responses to the questionnaire. Surprisingly, the model demonstrated a higher accuracy rate than initially anticipated, which was particularly impressive given the relatively small sample size involved in the study. The research's conclusion was unequivocal: Singaporean students responded favourably and engagedly to movie trailers than their Japanese peers. This finding highlights cultural differences in media reception and underscores the potential of targeted marketing strategies that cater to specific demographic and cultural preferences. Looking forward, the study's authors expressed a commitment to refining their research approach. They plan to enhance the questionnaire by testing more effectively formulated questions and exploring a broader array of machine-learning algorithms for better prediction accuracy. This ongoing improvement will likely provide deeper insights into the dynamics of audience engagement with media content across different cultures. This research, presented at the 9th IIAE International Conference, provided a detailed comparative analysis of how different student demographics perceive media content. It set the stage for future explorations into intelligent systems and image processing. The study offers valuable insights that could influence academic research and practical applications in media studies and marketing strategies by leveraging advanced data analysis techniques and machine learning.

Zafar and Kumar (2017) published that; the study's results showed significant improvements in various outcome measures for both treatment groups. These measures included pain severity assessed using the Visual Analog Scale (VAS), range of motion (ROM) for shoulder flexion, abduction, internal rotation, and external rotation, and pain and disability scores on the Shoulder Pain and Disability Index (SPADI). However, when comparing the two treatment groups, the laser therapy group exhibited more significant improvements than the ultrasound therapy group. Specifically, the laser therapy group showed mean differences that were, the range of motion (ROM) for shoulder flexion was found to be 2.94 times higher, while ROM for shoulder abduction was 5.45 times higher. Additionally, the SPADI pain score was 0.76 times higher, and the SPADI disability scores were 3.18 times higher. The study concluded that adding moist hot packs with either laser or ultrasound therapy effectively reduced pain, improved functional activity of the shoulder joints, and enhanced ROM in patients with grade 1 and 2 rotator cuff injuries. However, laser therapy was more effective than ultrasound therapy in managing these injuries. The research also mentioned various studies highlighting the benefits of heat therapy, ultrasound therapy, and low-level laser therapy in treating musculoskeletal conditions. These modalities effectively reduce pain, improve blood flow, increase tissue healing, and enhance range of motion in conditions such as muscle strains, hamstring tightness, periarthritis of shoulder, and osteoarthritis. For example, one study found that low-level laser therapy combined with exercise was more effective than exercise alone in treating subacromial syndrome, significantly improving pain and function. Another study showed that ultrasound therapy was effective in reducing pain and improving function in patients with rotator cuff tendinopathy. In conclusion, moist hot packs combined with laser or ultrasound therapy were found to be effective in reducing pain and improving functional activity in patients with grade 1 and 2 rotator cuff injuries. However, laser therapy showed superior results to ultrasound therapy in managing these injuries. The study acknowledged the limitation of a small sample size and recommended further research with a larger sample size and extended study duration to confirm these findings overall, this research highlights the potential benefits of using physical therapy modalities such as laser therapy and ultrasound therapy, in combination with heat therapy, for the conservative management of rotator cuff injuries. These non-invasive treatments can help alleviate pain, improve range of motion, and enhance function in affected patient's disorder.

As a summary, the research highlighted the VAS's ability to capture more nuanced emotional responses compared to traditional scales. Additionally, the study underscored the benefits of these therapies in managing musculoskeletal injuries, suggesting further research to validate their findings.

1.12.9 Effect of Range of Motion

Schlager et al., (2018) conducted a study to investigates the reliability of different methods used to assess joint hypermobility, a condition characterized by an increased range of motion (ROM) in multiple joints. The study focused on three specific assessment methods: the Beighton score (BES), the Contompasis score (CS), and the Hospital del Mar criteria (HdM). The researchers aimed to evaluate the consistency and accuracy of these methods by assessing their inter-rater (between different assessors) and intra-rater (within the same assessor) reliability. The study involved healthy adult participants and employed a test-retest design, where the assessments were conducted twice to measure reliability. The results showed that the total scores of the assessment methods and the majority of single-joint measurements (measured in degrees) had good-to-excellent reliability. This means that the scores were consistent across different assessors and within the same assessor, indicating that the methods are reliable for diagnosing generalized joint hypermobility (GJH). However, the study also found that some single-joint measurements needed better-to-moderate reliability, suggesting that assessing certain joints can be challenging and may lead to inconsistent results. To address this issue, the researchers emphasized the importance of using a structured protocol and standardized assessments when evaluating joint hypermobility. The structured protocol used in the study included detailed descriptions and illustrations of the starting positions, goniometer (an instrument used to measure angles) placement, anatomical landmarks, and stabilization of adjacent structures. This comprehensive approach aimed to ensure that the assessment of joint ROM in degrees was consistent and accurate across different assessors and settings. The study also highlighted the need for international consensus regarding GJH assessment methods and cut-off levels for hypermobility. There is yet to be a universally accepted standard for diagnosing GJH, which can lead to inconsistencies in diagnosis and treatment. By establishing a consensus, healthcare professionals can ensure that the assessment of GJH is based on reliable and valid methods, reducing the likelihood of false diagnoses and ensuring that individuals with GJH receive appropriate care. In conclusion, the research article provides valuable insights into the reliability of different hypermobility assessment methods. The findings demonstrate that the BeS, CS, and HdM methods have good-to-excellent reliability when used with a structured protocol and standardized assessments. However, the study also highlights the challenges in assessing certain joints and the need for further research to determine appropriate cut-off values for hypermobility. By establishing international consensus on GJH assessment methods and cut-off levels, healthcare professionals can improve the accuracy and consistency of GJH diagnoses, ultimately leading to better patient outcomes.

Walmsley et al., (2018) aims to provide evidence on the use of wearable sensors for calculating upper limb joint angles. The systematic review involved 66 studies that met the inclusion criteria out of 2191 records identified. It focused on the characteristics of commercial and custom wearable sensors, the populations for which researchers have adopted wearable sensors, and their established psychometric properties. The review revealed that both commercially available and custom wearable sensors have demonstrated evidence of validity, with errors of less than 5 degrees for all degrees of freedom at the wrist and elbow joints when compared to a robotic device. However, the range in error is greater when measured in vivo and compared to a pseudo-gold standard. The study concluded that wearable sensors have the potential to be viable instruments for measuring joint angles in the upper limb during active movement. Still, it highlighted the need for additional research and standardization to guide clinical application. The review found that wearable sensors offer portability, usability, size, and cost advantages compared to laboratory-based 3DMA systems. It also highlighted the limitations of traditional measurement tools such as goniometers, which are limited to measuring joint angles in single planes and static positions, and 3DMA systems, which are immobile, expensive, and require considerable expertise. The document outlined the wearable sensors' calibration methods, including system and static anatomical calibration, and emphasized the importance of calibration and angle calculation methods for achieving sufficient accuracy. The systematic review also detailed the characteristics and placement of wearable sensors, including commercial and custom brands, dimensions, components used, and sampling rates. It identified the variations in placement, calibration methods, and fusion algorithms, which were shown to influence accuracy. Additionally, the document presented the populations for whom researchers have applied wearable sensors and how they have been used, shedding light on the diverse applications of wearable sensors in measuring joint angles in the upper limb. In conclusion, the systematic review provides valuable insights into the potential of wearable sensors for measuring upper limb joint angles. It emphasizes the need for further research, standardization, and calibration to ensure the accuracy and reliability of these sensors for clinical application. The findings of this review have implications for clinicians and researchers seeking accurate and reliable measurement tools for assessing upper limb range of motion in various clinical populations, including those with orthopaedic, musculoskeletal, and neurological disorders.

As a conclusion, the study found good-to-excellent reliability for the methods overall, although certain single-joint measurements showed moderate reliability. Moreover, the study highlighted the advantages of wearable sensors, such as portability and cost, over traditional tools like goniometers and 3DMA systems. However, it stressed the need for further research, standardization, and improved calibration methods to enhance sensor accuracy for clinical applications in populations with musculoskeletal or neurological disorders.

1.12.10 Effect of DASH Outcome Measure

Hardy et al. (2019) stated that, the study investigated the impact of various factors on shoulder outcome measures in asymptomatic individuals, revealing several important findings: health perception significantly affects shoulder function scores, The study found that an individual's perception of their overall health significantly impacted their Disability of the Arm, Shoulder, and Hand (DASH) score. Those who reported better overall health tended to have improved shoulder function scores. This highlights the importance of considering a patient's general health status when interpreting shoulder outcome measures. Secondly, Sex and hand dominance influence shoulder scores: The research revealed that sex and hand dominance affected the scores of the American Shoulder and Elbow Surgeons Standard Shoulder Assessment (ASES) and Constant measures. These demographic factors should be taken into account when evaluating shoulder function and comparing scores across different patient populations. Development of prediction models: The study developed prediction models to estimate shoulder outcome scores based on Sex, hand dominance, and overall health perception. These models can help clinicians provide more personalized care and set realistic expectations for patients. Realistic expectations for outcome measures: An important finding of the study was that achieving the highest possible scores on shoulder outcome measures may only be realistic for some patients, even in asymptomatic individuals. This challenges the notion that perfect scores should be the goal for all patients and emphasizes the need for individualized assessment and treatment planning. Importance of comprehensive assessment: The study highlighted the significance of using health-specific measures alongside shoulder outcome measures to provide a more comprehensive understanding of a patient's health status. This approach can lead to more accurate assessments and better-tailored treatment plans. Individualized healthcare: The research emphasized the importance of gathering demographic information and considering individual factors when interpreting shoulder outcome scores. This supports the trend towards more personalized healthcare and the need for clinicians to consider multiple factors when assessing patient progress. Implications for clinical practice: The findings suggest that clinicians should interpret shoulder outcome measure scores in the context of various demographic factors and overall health status. This may lead to more accurate assessments of patient progress and more effective treatment planning. Potential for improved patient communication: Understanding the influence of factors like health perception, Sex, and hand dominance on shoulder scores can help clinicians better explain results to patients and set realistic expectations for treatment outcomes. The study opens up avenues for further research into the development and refinement of prediction models for shoulder outcome measures and investigations into other factors that may influence these scores. The research highlights potential limitations in current shoulder outcome measures, suggesting that they may need to fully capture the complexity of individual patient experiences and factors affecting shoulder function. In conclusion, this study provides valuable insights into the factors influencing shoulder outcome measures in asymptomatic individuals. By considering health perception, Sex, hand dominance, and other demographic factors, clinicians can provide more personalized and effective care to patients with shoulder conditions. The development of prediction models and the emphasis on comprehensive assessment techniques may lead to improved patient outcomes and more accurate evaluations of treatment effectiveness in the field of shoulder care.

Ogura et al, (2021) conducted a study, a multifaceted approach was employed to investigate the Disabilities of the Arm, Shoulder, and Hand (DASH) outcome measure following essential upper extremity tumour surgery. The research, which encompassed various key elements, provided valuable insights into the relationship between patient-reported changes and DASH scores, as well as the measure's discriminative ability in this specific context. The study's findings were presented through a series of visual and tabular representations, each offering a unique perspective on the data. One of the central components was a set of box-and-whiskers plots, illustrated in Figure 2, which effectively demonstrated the correlation between changes in DASH scores and patients' responses to anchor questions. This visual representation served as a crucial tool in understanding how patients' subjective assessments of their condition aligned with the more objective DASH scoring system. Further bolstering the study's analytical depth was the inclusion of a Receiver Operating Characteristic (ROC) curve, presented in Figure 3. This curve plotted the true positive rate (sensitivity) against the false-positive rate (1-specificity) for the DASH questionnaire scores. The resulting Area Under the Curve (AUC) of 0.75 indicated a good discriminative ability of the model, reinforcing the DASH questionnaire's validity as an assessment tool in the context of upper extremity tumour surgery. The researchers also provided a comprehensive overview of patient demographics and baseline characteristics in Table I. This information included details such as age, sex, histologic diagnosis, and the type of surgery the participants underwent. Such data is crucial for contextualizing the study's findings and understanding the population to which the results may be most applicable. Complementing this demographic information, Table II offered a detailed breakdown of DASH scores, anchor questions, and the changes in DASH scores observed throughout the study. This table was particularly valuable in highlighting the distribution of responses to anchor questions and the mean changes in DASH scores. It provided a nuanced view of how patients' conditions evolved and how these changes were reflected in their DASH scores. One of the study's most significant contributions was the comparison of Minimal Clinically Important Differences (MCID) and DASH scores among various orthopaedic conditions, presented in Table III. This comparative analysis included MCID calculations from different studies and specifically highlighted the MCID values for patients undergoing surgery for upper limb tumours in the current series. By situating their findings within the broader context of orthopaedic research, the authors provided a valuable frame of reference for interpreting their results. The integration of these various elements – from visual representations to detailed tabular data – allowed for a comprehensive and nuanced understanding of the DASH outcome measure's effectiveness in the context of upper extremity tumour surgery. By examining the relationship between patient-reported changes and DASH scores, assessing the measure's discriminative ability, and comparing their findings to those in other orthopaedic conditions, Ogura et al. have made a significant contribution to the field. Their work not only validates the use of the DASH questionnaire in this specific context but also provides valuable insights that can inform future research and clinical practice in the management of upper extremity tumours.

As a summary, the study developed prediction models to estimate shoulder outcome scores based on these factors, emphasizing the importance of setting realistic expectations and individualized care. It also highlighted the need for comprehensive assessments, incorporating health-specific measures, to better tailor treatment plans and improve patient communication. Additionally, their study, which included patient demographics and changes in DASH scores, validated the DASH tool's effectiveness for assessing outcomes in this context and provided valuable insights into its application in upper extremity tumor surgery.

11.2 RESEARCH GAP

The management of shoulder periarthritis remains a complex and debated topic within the field of rehabilitation. While various treatment modalities have been proposed, there is a significant divergence of opinion regarding the most effective approaches and the optimal order in which to implement them. Recent studies have highlighted Modified Posterior Shoulder Stretching as an effective management strategy for addressing Glenohumeral Internal Rotation Deficit (GIRD) and Posterior Shoulder Tightness (PST). Türksan and Yesilyaprak (2023) emphasize the efficacy of this technique in improving shoulder function, suggesting that it plays a crucial role in the rehabilitation of patients with these specific conditions. Furthermore, evidence supports the use of end-range mobilizations at the glenohumeral joint as a proven method for enhancing range of motion in patients suffering from Adhesive Capsulitis. Research conducted by S. Naureen (2022) demonstrates that such mobilizations can lead to significant improvements in shoulder mobility, thereby alleviating pain and enhancing functional outcomes. These findings underscore the importance of targeted interventions in managing shoulder pathologies.

Despite the existing evidence supporting these treatment modalities, there remains a notable gap in the literature regarding direct comparisons between different therapeutic techniques. Specifically, there is a lack of studies investigating the effectiveness of Modified Posterior Capsular Stretching versus Grade 3 Maitland Mobilization for patients with shoulder periarthritis. This gap is critical, as understanding how these techniques compare could inform clinical practice and guide rehabilitation protocols. The absence of comparative research limits clinicians' ability to make evidence-based decisions regarding treatment selection for shoulder periarthritis. As such, further investigation is warranted to evaluate the relative effectiveness of these two interventions. By addressing this research gap, future studies could provide valuable insights that enhance treatment strategies and improve patient outcomes in individuals suffering from shoulder-related disorders.

In conclusion, while current literature supports various effective techniques for managing shoulder conditions, the lack of comparative studies specifically focusing on Modified Posterior Capsular Stretching and Grade 3 Maitland Mobilization represents an important area for future research. Addressing this gap will be essential for advancing our understanding of optimal treatment approaches for shoulder periarthritis and ensuring that patients receive the most effective care possible.

1.13 AIMS

- To evaluate the effectiveness of Modified Posterior Capsular Stretching VS Grade 3 Maitland Mobilization Among Patients with Periarthritis Shoulder by using range of motion, visual analogue scale (VAS) and DASH questionnaire as an outcome measure to find out the result.

1.14 OBJECTIVES

1.14.1 General objectives

- To find out the Effectiveness of Modified Posterior Capsular Stretching VS Grade 3 Maitland Mobilization Among Patients with Periarthritis Shoulder

1.14.2 Specific objectives

- To compare the Effectiveness of Modified Posterior Capsular Stretching Vs Grade 3 Maitland Mobilization on pain among patients with periarthritis shoulder.
- To compare the Effectiveness of Modified Posterior Capsular Stretching Vs Grade 3 Maitland Mobilization on range of motion among patients with periarthritis shoulder.
- To compare the Effectiveness of Modified Posterior Capsular Stretching Vs Grade 3 Maitland Mobilization on functional ability among patients with periarthritis shoulder.

1.15 HYPOTHESIS

1.15.1 Null Hypothesis

- There is a no significant differences in the effect of modified posterior capsular stretching in reducing pain, improving range of motion and improving functional ability among patients with periarthritis shoulder
- There is a no significant differences in the effect of grade 3 Maitland Mobilization in reducing pain, improving range of motion and improving functional ability among patients with periarthritis shoulder.

1.15.2 Alternative Hypothesis

- There is a significant difference in the effect of modified posterior capsular stretching in reducing pain, improving range of motion and improving functional ability among patients with periarthritis shoulder
- There is a significant difference in the effect of grade 3 Maitland Mobilization in reducing pain, improving range of motion and functional ability among patients with periarthritis shoulder.

CHAPTER 2

MATERIALS AND METHODS

2.1 Study Design

The present investigation adopts a single-blind, quasi-experimental approach, comparing two groups of interventions. The chosen design stems from the objectives of the research and insights from data collection. In this study's single-blind format, participants remain unaware of which intervention they receive, though the researchers or evaluators do have this knowledge. Quasi-experimental research differs from its experimental counterpart in that participant assignment to treatment groups isn't random, but rather based on comparing the impact of two different treatments against each other. Assessments are conducted at two time points: initially to establish a baseline before any treatment, and again at the end of a fourth-week period. This approach allows for the analysis of shifts in the dependent variables over time across the treatment cohorts. By employing blinding, the study design aims to make reliable comparisons between the outcomes of the two treatments and mitigate potential biases.

When conducting full-scale trials is impractical due to constraints like budget, time, ethical considerations, or political hurdles, quasi-experimental designs are frequently adopted as a preferred alternative. Compared to traditional trials, these quasi-experimental methods come with their set of advantages. One such advantage is the diminution of interference with the natural setting of the intervention, which, in turn, enhances the generalizability or external validity of the results. Another benefit is mitigating issues related to internal validity that could arise from the participants' reactions to being assigned to control or treatment groups. Quasi-experiments, therefore, serve as a viable option, offering a balance between the rigorous control of experimental designs and the real-world relevance that comes from observing outcomes in less contrived settings. While they may not provide the same level of causal certainty as randomized controlled trials, their design is often sophisticated enough to yield valuable insights. This is particularly relevant in scenarios where traditional experiments are challenging and infeasible. The adaptability of quasi-experiments is another aspect that makes them appealing; these designs can be tailored to fit a variety of situations and contexts, including those that are dynamic and evolving. This flexibility is essential when researchers aim to understand phenomena within their natural environments. Consequently, quasi-experimental designs are pivotal in research fields where authentic contexts are paramount for relevant insights. In summary, although quasi-experiments may be second to randomized trials in the hierarchy of research design rigour, they represent an indispensable tool in the researcher's toolkit. Their application is particularly valued when facing practical barriers to conducting traditional experiments, and their strategic use can lead to meaningful contributions to knowledge, especially in fields where situational authenticity is critical. Lavis et al., (2017)

2.2 Study Population

The study centered on individuals seeking care at the AIMST Physio Clinic within AIMST University in Bedong, Kedah. A meticulous screening was conducted to guarantee the study's accuracy and dependability. Only volunteers matching designated qualifications were included in the study, which might have included specific considerations such as the duration and severity of shoulder pain and a commitment to participate actively in the research.

Participants who qualified were directed to the AIMST Physio Clinic at AIMST University in Bedong, Kedah, where they reported symptoms of periarthritis of the shoulder. The aim of collecting this information was to secure relevant data. The study objective to evaluate the relative effectiveness of modified posterior capsular stretching versus grade 3 Maitland mobilization in patients with periarthritis of the shoulder treated at the AIMST Physio Clinic, AIMST University, Bedong Kedah. Participants were carefully chosen based on their industry relevance and conformity with established criteria to achieve this.

2.3 Study Duration with Ethical Approval

The study was carried out from June to July 2024 at the AIMST Physio Clinic, located within AIMST University in Bedong, Kedah. The Research Ethics Committee of AIMST University provided ethical approval for this research. The investigation was structured as an assessor-blind non-randomised controlled trial, with the ethical approval code AUHEC/FAHP/11/06/2024/2.

2.4 Study Setting

The research focused on individuals undergoing treatment at the AIMST Physio Clinic, a facility situated within AIMST University's campus in Bedong, Kedah. This clinic served as the primary site for patient recruitment and data collection for the study.

2.5 Sample Size and Sample Selection

The study's sample size was calculated using Epi Info Statistical Software, developed by Dean and Andrew G. in 2000. This software considers several key factors to determine an appropriate sample size, including the overall population size, the desired margin of error, and the statistical power of the study. According to this software, sample size given is 80 parameters were set. This sample size ensures that the study has sufficient statistical power to detect meaningful effects while maintaining a reasonable margin of error.

2.6 Sampling Technique

The clinical trial initially recruited 90 participants. These participants were then randomly divided into two experimental groups of 45 patients each. The first group (Group 1) received a treatment protocol consisting of Hot Pack Application combined with Modified Posterior Capsular Stretching. The second group (Group 2) underwent a treatment regimen involving Hot Pack Application followed by Grade 3 Maitland Mobilization Technique. To evaluate the effectiveness of these interventions, the study incorporated both pre- and post-intervention assessments. These assessments focused on measuring pain levels and shoulder range of motion and functional ability by using validated tools, specifically the Visual Analog Scale (VAS) for pain and a goniometer for range of motion measurements and DASH Outcome measure questionnaire for functional ability.

2.7 Selection of Criteria

The study recruited 90 patients diagnosed with periarthritis shoulder, based on referrals from physicians. These participants, comprising both men and women, were aged between 40 and 60 years and were originally patients at AIMST University. To ensure informed participation, each potential participant received an informational booklet that outlined the study's objectives in detail. The researchers then applied specific inclusion criteria to determine eligibility for the study. These criteria were designed to ensure a suitable and representative sample for the research.

2.7.1 Inclusion Criteria

The study employed specific eligibility criteria for participant selection. These inclusion requirements were as follows:

- Patients who are Medically diagnosed cases of Periarthritis Shoulder
- Pain and stiffness over shoulder joint
- Age group above 40 – 60 years
- Patient in frozen stage
- Tested positive in Apley's scratch test
- Both males and females were included
- Diabetes patients with controlled
- Willing to participate

2.7.2 Exclusion Criteria

The criteria for exclusion were:

- Any shoulder surgery, fractures, dislocation or stroke
- Pregnant or lactating females
- History of previous periarthritis shoulder treatment
- Systemic inflammation or osteoarthritis in other joints

2.7.3 Theoretical Support for Inclusion Criteria

This criterion ensures that all participants have given their informed consent to be part of the study. It is crucial for ethical reasons and ensures that participants are aware of the study's purpose, procedures, potential risks, and benefits. Participants must voluntarily agree to join the study without any coercion. Furthermore, this criterion indicates that the study is open to all genders, ensuring a diverse and representative sample. Including both males and females helps in understanding how the condition and its treatment may affect different genders. Moreover, Visual Analogue scale (VAS) is a tool used to measure pain intensity. It typically ranges from 0 (no pain) to 10 (worst possible pain). This criterion requires that participants have a pain score of at least 1 until 4, indicating moderate pain to less pain. This ensures that the participants have a significant level of pain that warrants intervention and study. Not only that, this criterion specifies that the condition must be present in only one shoulder. This is important for consistency in the study, as having bilateral periarthritis could complicate the assessment and treatment outcomes. More than other, focusing on unilateral cases allows for more precise measurement of the intervention's effects on the affected shoulder. Finally, this criterion specifies that only individuals who have been experiencing symptoms for more than three months are eligible. This duration ensures that the condition is chronic and not in the acute phase, which is important for the study's objectives. Jain and Shukla (2023). By adhering to these inclusion criteria, the study aims to select a specific group of participants who are most likely to benefit from and contribute valuable data to the research. This careful selection helps in achieving reliable and valid results. In a phase often referred to as the "frozen" stage, individuals experience a notable reduction in pain accompanied by a significant increase in stiffness. During this period, the shoulder capsule undergoes fibrosis, leading to a restriction in the range of motion, particularly affecting external rotation. This limitation can severely impact daily activities and overall mobility. Typically, this stage persists for a duration of four to twelve months, during which patients may find it challenging to perform tasks that require shoulder movement. Understanding this phase is crucial for effective management and rehabilitation of shoulder conditions. Berner et al. (2024). Research suggests that diabetes may play a role in the development of frozen shoulder, primarily through glycation and inflammatory processes. These mechanisms can lead to capsular fibrosis, resulting in the tightening and contracture of the shoulder joint. To assess whether diabetes is a potential cause of frozen shoulder, it is crucial to establish a temporal relationship between the onset of diabetes and the occurrence of frozen shoulder symptoms. While demonstrating this relationship is important, it may not be sufficient on its own to confirm a direct causal link. Gaining a deeper understanding of how diabetes and frozen shoulder are interconnected could provide valuable insights into their underlying mechanisms. This knowledge could ultimately inform more effective treatment and management strategies for individuals suffering from both conditions, enhancing their quality of life and recovery outcomes. Further research in this area is essential to clarify these associations and improve patient care. (Dyer BP et al.,2023)

2.7.4 Theoretical Support for Exclusion Criteria

Pregnant and breastfeeding women are often excluded from clinical trials and certain medical treatments due to potential risks to the fetus or infant. These risks include teratogenic effects (birth defects caused by exposure to certain substances) and adverse reactions that could affect the developing baby or the breastfeeding infant. Historically, this exclusion was aimed at protecting the health of both the mother and child, but it has also led to a lack of data on the safety and efficacy of many treatments for this population. Furthermore, Patients who have undergone shoulder surgery are excluded from certain studies or treatments to avoid confounding variables that could affect the outcomes. Previous shoulder surgeries can alter the anatomy and biomechanics of the shoulder, potentially influencing the effectiveness of treatments being studied. Additionally, prior surgeries might lead to implications or adverse events that could skew study results. Plus, any impact from humerus fractures, dislocation, or cerebrovascular accident These underlying conditions can significantly influence the progression and treatment response of periarthritis shoulder, making it difficult to isolate the effects of the treatment being studied. For instance, the pathophysiology and recovery trajectory of periarthritis shoulder due to trauma or neurological events can differ markedly from idiopathic periarthritis shoulder. Mertens et al. (2022)

Moreover, patients who have previously received treatment for periarthritis of shoulder are excluded to ensure that the study population is homogeneous and to avoid confounding variables. Previous treatments can influence the natural course of the condition and the response to new interventions, making it difficult to isolate the effects of the treatment being studied. This exclusion helps in maintaining the integrity of the study results by ensuring that all participants are experiencing their condition for the first time and have not been influenced by prior interventions. And finally, patients with systemic inflammation or osteoarthritis in other joints are excluded because these conditions can affect the study outcomes. Systemic inflammation, such as that seen in rheumatoid arthritis or other autoimmune diseases, can complicate the clinical picture and influence the response to treatment. Similarly, osteoarthritis in other joints can lead to generalized pain and mobility issues, which could confound the assessment of shoulder-specific treatments. By excluding these patients, researchers aim to create a more controlled environment where the effects of the treatment on periarthritis of shoulder can be more accurately measured. Haider et al. (2022)

2.8 Tools and Materials

2.8.1 Pain Scale

Visual Analogue Scale (VAS)

Visual Analogue Scale (VAS) as outcome measure, Hayes and Patterson introduced the visual analog scale (VAS) to assess pain in 1921. A single handwritten mark, put at a single position along a 10-cm line, symbolizes a continuum between the two extremes of the scale "no pain" on the left end (0 cm) and "worst pain" on the right end (10 cm) is used to record self-reported assessments of symptoms. The patient's pain is measured in centimeters, beginning at the left end of the scale and going to their markers. The data may be used to compare pain amongst patients with comparable diseases or to monitor a patient's pain as it progresses. The scale has also been used to assess ambulation, mood, hunger, asthma, dyspepsia, and pain. Despite contradictory data regarding its superiority over other techniques, the VAS is still widely used in professional and domestic settings for recording pain. Delgado et al., (2018)

2.8.2 Range of Motion

Goniometer

The assessment of range of motion is a fundamental aspect of physical therapy assessments, commonly referred to as goniometry. In the context of musculoskeletal disorders, mastering the technique of goniometry is seen as an indispensable skill for clinicians. This method of measurement yields data that can confirm or rule out functional impairments in the normal movement of the body's joints. By accurately gauging ROM, clinicians can create and document clear evidence to demonstrate the impact and efficacy of various treatment interventions. In clinical settings, the precise quantification of ROM serves as a crucial criterion for treatment outcomes. It provides objective insights into a patient's progress, verifying the success of therapeutic methods, and helping tailor ongoing care plans. The information gathered through ROM assessments helps to guide treatment choices, ensuring that therapy is targeted and appropriate to the patient's specific condition. Goniometry is not just a tool for diagnosis and evaluation it also plays a crucial role in the development of treatment protocols. When applied correctly, it helps in charting the course of rehabilitation, setting benchmarks for improvement, and in many cases, motivating patients by presenting tangible progress in their functional abilities. Moreover, ROM measurements collected via goniometry are valuable in constructing a body of evidence to support the effectiveness of physical therapy treatments. Such data can be used in research studies to further understand musculoskeletal disorders and to refine therapeutic techniques. Ultimately, goniometry is not just a tool for individual patient assessment but a means of advancing the overall knowledge and effectiveness of physical therapy practices. Elgendy and El-Khalek (2019)

In orthopedic surgery and physical therapy, goniometers have become standard tools for gauging the angles at which joints can bend. However, the precision of the shorter versions of these devices is debatable, especially when we consider the long bones, such as the femur, involved in knee motion. With technological advancements, smartphones can host various applications that utilize built-in accelerometers to approximate joint angles. This development has sparked numerous research endeavors to evaluate their precision, yielding multiple outcomes. A need marks the quest for the most effective method for joint angle measurement for a tool that is consistent and reliable across multiple evaluations and observers and showcases a low margin of error. Ease of use and the ability to quickly obtain measurements in the dynamic environment of an outpatient clinic is also critically important. While radiographic imaging has been deemed the benchmark for measuring angles, its practicality is hindered by operational costs, patient exposure to radiation, and its questionable capacity for detecting incremental changes in a joint's range of motion. In recognizing the limitations posed by traditional radiographs, the healthcare field is actively exploring the acceptable margins of error across devices suitable for everyday clinical applications to ascertain which offers the most significant benefits. The intention is to identify a measurement tool that provides high accuracy and seamless clinical integration, effectively balancing precision and practicality. This pursuit significantly enhances the selection of effective treatment plans while also contributing to the body of research by ensuring that the data collected are reliable and replicable across different settings and scenarios. Hancock et al. (2018)

2.8.3 DASH Outcome Measure

The DASH (Disabilities of the Arm, Shoulder and Hand) scoring system has demonstrated a significant association with degenerative pathologies, largely due to its comprehensive approach to upper extremity assessment. This association stems from the DASH's ability to evaluate function across the entire upper limb, including the shoulder, elbow, and wrist. Such a holistic approach is particularly valuable when dealing with degenerative shoulder conditions, which often have far-reaching effects on adjacent joints and overall upper limb function. The DASH's broad scope allows for a more thorough evaluation of a patient's condition and functional status. This is especially crucial in cases of degenerative pathologies, where the impact may extend beyond the primary site of concern. By assessing function across multiple joints, the DASH provides a more complete picture of the patient's upper extremity capabilities and limitations. Moreover, the DASH has proven particularly useful in cases of traumatic injuries that affect multiple areas of the upper extremity. Its design enables clinicians to assess function across various joints, making it an invaluable tool when injuries extend beyond the shoulder. This versatility sets the DASH apart from more localized assessment tools, allowing for a more comprehensive evaluation of complex upper limb conditions. The DASH's effectiveness in assessing degenerative shoulder conditions, combined with its broader applicability to the entire upper limb, makes it a preferred choice for many researchers and clinicians. This comprehensive approach enables more accurate and thorough evaluations of upper extremity pathologies and treatments. The selection of appropriate outcome measures is crucial in both research and clinical practice. The DASH's unique characteristics make it suitable for a wide range of upper extremity evaluations, offering a more holistic assessment compared to joint-specific measures. This versatility can guide healthcare professionals in choosing the most appropriate scoring system for their specific needs, ultimately leading to more precise and comprehensive evaluations of upper extremity conditions and treatment outcomes. Ashton et al. (2020)

The Disabilities of the Arm, Shoulder and Hand (DASH) outcome measure is a comprehensive tool designed to assess upper limb functioning. This instrument consists of 30 items, each scored on a scale from 1 to 5, providing a nuanced evaluation of a patient's condition. The DASH's scoring methodology is both flexible and robust, allowing for the calculation of a total score even when some items are incomplete, provided that at least 27 of the 30 items have been answered. To enhance interpretability and standardization, the DASH employs an algorithm that converts the raw scores into a standardized scale ranging from 0 to 100. This conversion process also incorporates a method for handling missing values, ensuring that incomplete responses do not invalidate the entire assessment. The resulting standardized score offers a clear and easily comparable measure of upper limb function across different patients or time points. The DASH's 30 items are carefully crafted to capture a holistic picture of upper limb functioning. This includes assessments of pain levels, which can significantly impact a patient's quality of life and ability to perform tasks. Additionally, the questionnaire evaluates various activities of daily living, providing insight into how the patient's condition affects their everyday functioning and independence. Recognizing the need for a more concise assessment tool in certain clinical or research settings, a shortened version of the DASH, known as the QuickDASH, has been developed. This abbreviated form consists of 11 items selected from the full DASH questionnaire. The QuickDASH maintains a similar scoring approach to its parent instrument, allowing for rapid assessment while still providing valuable insights into upper limb function. In research settings, the QuickDASH can be derived from completed full DASH questionnaires, offering flexibility in data analysis and reporting. This allows researchers to compare results using both the comprehensive DASH and the more focused QuickDASH, potentially providing additional perspectives on the data. The DASH and QuickDASH represent valuable tools in the assessment of upper limb function, offering clinicians and researchers standardized, reliable methods for evaluating patients with various upper extremity conditions. Their ability to quantify both pain and functional aspects provides a comprehensive view of a patient's status, facilitating treatment planning and outcome measurement. Prodinger et al. (2019)

2.9 Procedure of the Study

2.9.1 Data Collection

The study's data collection process began with informal conversations between researchers and potential participants, designed to create a comfortable and trusting atmosphere. Participant recruitment strictly adhered to predefined inclusion and exclusion criteria. After successful screening, each participant provided signed informed consent. Researchers emphasized the protection of personal information throughout the study. To ensure confidentiality, only anonymized data was published, with all personal identifiers omitted. Data access and analysis were restricted to the lead investigator. This approach prioritized participant privacy while maintaining research integrity and compliance with ethical standards.

The research policy strictly mandates that participants' personal information is not disclosed in any publications. Before any data is published, it is crucial to obtain all necessary licenses and consents. Researchers provided participants with a thorough explanation of the study's details, including the methodology, the significance of consistent attendance, the potential positive outcomes, and the participants' right to withdraw from the study at any time. This comprehensive briefing ensured that participants were fully informed about their involvement and the study's objectives. Participants were made aware of several potential benefits of their involvement in the study. These benefits included the opportunity to contribute to scientific progress, which can have far-reaching implications for future research and healthcare practices. Additionally, participants were encouraged to actively engage in their own healthcare, fostering a sense of empowerment and personal responsibility.

Participation in the study offered a unique opportunity for individuals to engage in intellectually stimulating activities. This aspect of the research was designed to be both enriching and rewarding, providing participants with mental challenges that could contribute to their cognitive well-being. The intellectual engagement inherent in the study procedures and assessments was seen as a valuable benefit, potentially enhancing participants' mental acuity and knowledge base. A key advantage of participation was the access to exceptional healthcare services provided by renowned experts in the field. This high-quality care was offered at no cost to the participants, representing a significant benefit, especially for those who might not otherwise have access to such specialized medical attention. The opportunity to receive care from leading professionals in a research setting was highlighted as a rare and valuable experience.

The study's interventions and assessments were carefully designed to provide comprehensive insights into participants' health. These procedures had the potential to uncover valuable information about individual health status, offering participants a deeper understanding of their physical condition. Such knowledge could be instrumental in informing future healthcare decisions and practices. Furthermore, participants were informed about the potential for improving their overall well-being and quality of life through their involvement in the study. The research team emphasized that the interventions and regular health assessments could lead to enhanced physical and mental health outcomes. This holistic approach to health improvement was presented as a significant potential benefit of participation. The combination of intellectual stimulation, access to expert healthcare, and the potential for health improvements created a compelling case for participation. Researchers stressed that while the primary goal of the study was to advance scientific knowledge, the personal benefits to participants could be substantial. These benefits extended beyond the immediate scope of the study, potentially influencing participants' long-term health and well-being. By highlighting these multifaceted benefits, the research team aimed to demonstrate the value of participation beyond the contribution to scientific progress. This approach not only served to motivate potential participants but also underscored the ethical commitment to ensuring that research subjects derive tangible benefits from their involvement in scientific studies.

In this study, participants were randomly assigned to one of two treatment groups, with all individuals blinded to their group allocation to minimize bias. The first group (Group 1) received a combination therapy of modified posterior capsule stretching and hot pack treatment. In contrast, the second group (Group 2) was administered grade 3 Maitland mobilization alongside hot pack treatment. The intervention schedule was consistent across both groups, with participants engaging in treatment sessions once daily, three times per week, for a total duration of four weeks. This structured approach ensured uniformity in treatment frequency and duration across all participants. To evaluate the effectiveness of these interventions, the study incorporated both pre- and post-intervention assessments. These assessments focused on two key parameters: pain levels and shoulder range of motion in stationary patients. To ensure accuracy and reliability in data collection, the researchers employed validated measurement tools. Specifically, the Visual Analog Scale (VAS) was used to assess pain intensity, while a goniometer was utilized to measure shoulder range of motion and DASH outcome measure is used to evaluate functional ability. This comprehensive assessment protocol, combined with the blinded, randomized group allocation and consistent treatment schedule, was designed to provide robust and reliable data on the comparative efficacy of the two intervention approaches in managing shoulder-related issues.

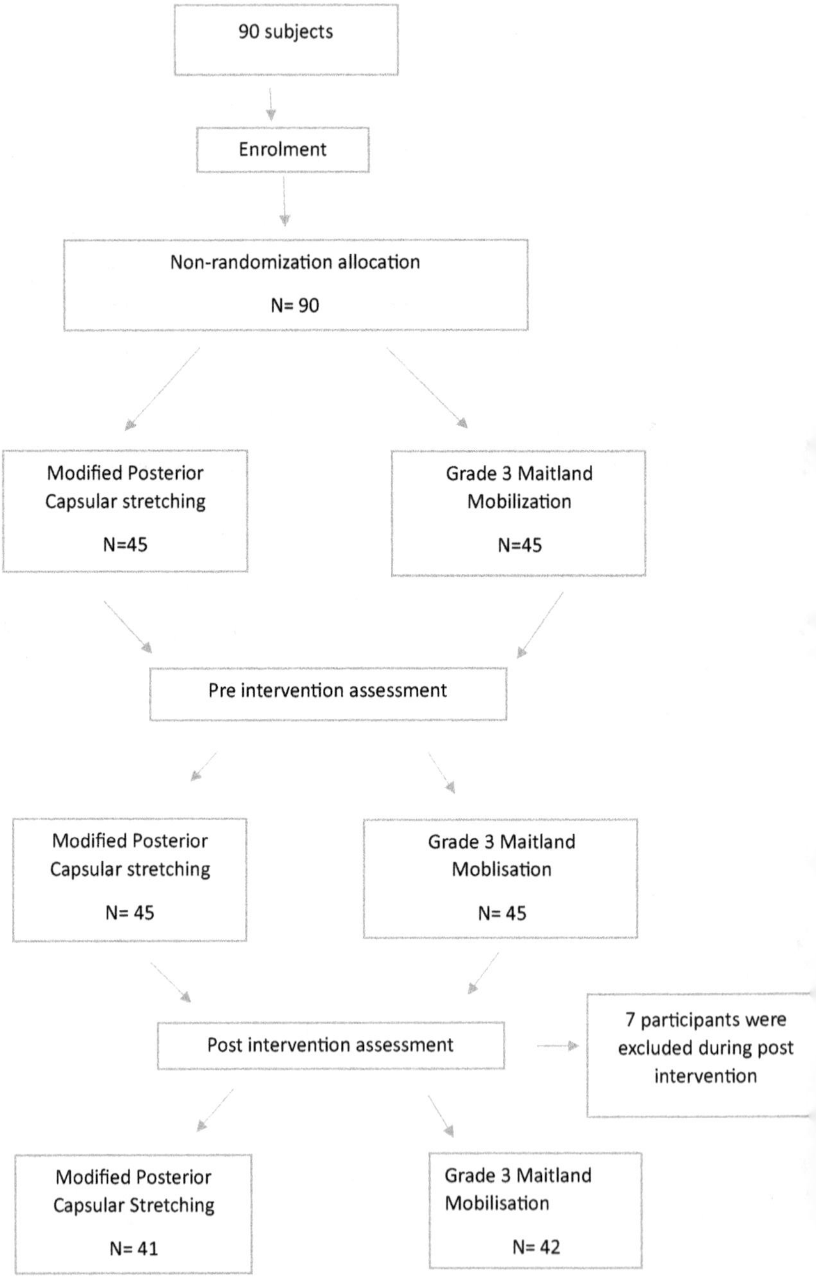

Figure 3: Participant Recruitment and Group Assignment Flowchart

2.9.2 Modified Posterior Capsular Stretching Protocol

Hot Pack Protocol

Perform moist hot pack for 10 minutes in supine-lying position.

Modified Posterior Capsular Stretching Protocol [Tahran and Yesilyaprak (2020)]

The modified posterior capsule stretching exercise is performed with the patient in a side-lying position. This positioning is crucial as it helps to restrict scapular abduction, ensuring that the stretch targets the intended area effectively. To begin, the patient aligns their forearms, with the arm of the non-affected side placed on top of the affected arm. This alignment is important as it limits the external rotation of the humerus on the affected side, focusing the stretch on the posterior capsule. Using the opposite (top) arm, the patient gently moves the affected arm's humerus into horizontal adduction. This movement should be controlled and deliberate, avoiding any sudden or jerky motions. The stretch is held for a duration of 30 seconds. This is repeated 5 times, constituting one complete set. The extended hold time allows for an effective stretch of the posterior capsule tissues. As per the protocol outlined by Tahran and Yesilyaprak (2020) this exercise regimen is to be performed once daily, three days per week, for a total duration of four weeks. This consistent schedule is designed to promote gradual improvement in shoulder flexibility and function while allowing adequate rest between sessions. It's important that patients perform this exercise with proper technique and adhere to the prescribed frequency to maximize its therapeutic benefits while minimizing the risk of overexertion or injury.

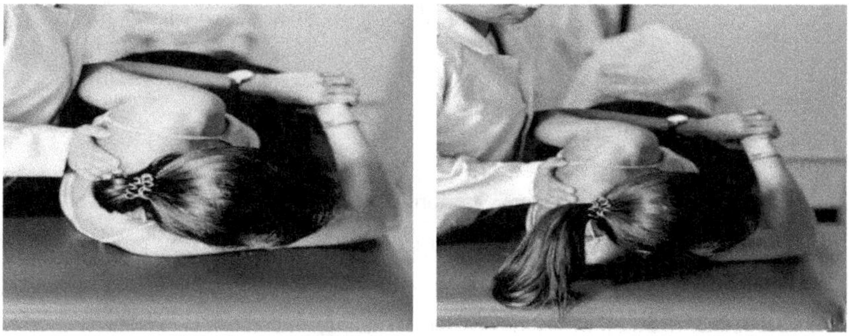

Fig. 4: Modified Posterior Capsular Stretching Protocol

2.9.3 Grade 3 Maitland Mobilization Protocol

Hot Pack Protocol

Perform moist hot pack for 10 minutes in supine-lying position.

Glenohumeral Caudal Glide [Kisner et al. (2017)]

Patient Positioning:

The patient lies supine (on their back) with the affected arm in a relaxed position. The forearm is supported between the trunk and elbow, ensuring comfort and stability.

Therapist's Hand Placement:

The therapist positions one hand in the patient's axilla (armpit) for support and control. The web space (area between thumb and index finger) of the therapist's other hand is carefully placed just distal to the acromion process of the scapula.

Mobilization Technique:

Using the hand placed near the acromion, the therapist applies a mobilizing force, gently gliding the humerus in an inferior direction (downward towards the feet).

Oscillation and Stretch Application:

The therapist initiates the technique with a sustained stretch force lasting a minimum of 6 seconds. The therapist then repeats this process with slow, rhythmic stretches at 3-4 second intervals.

Treatment Schedule:

This mobilization technique is performed once daily, with three sessions per week, over a 4-week intervention period. This consistent application allows for progressive improvement while providing adequate rest between sessions. The Grade 3 Maitland mobilization, combined with this specific protocol, aims to improve joint mobility, reduce pain, and enhance overall shoulder function in patients with shoulder conditions.

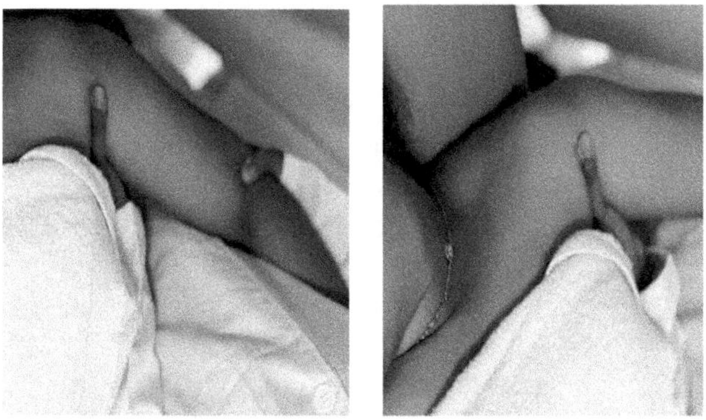

Fig 5: Glenohumeral Caudal Glide

Glenohumeral Anterior Glide [Kisner et al. (2017)]

Patient Positioning:

Prone with arm resting position over the edge of the treatment table, supported on the therapist's thigh and stabilize the acromion.

Therapist's Hand Placement:

Stand facing the top of the table with the leg closer to the table in a forward stride position. Support the patient's arm against thigh with other hand.

Mobilization Technique:

Using the hand placed near the acromion, the therapist applies a mobilizing force, gently gliding the humerus in an inferior direction (downward towards the feet).

Oscillation and Stretch Application:

The therapist initiates the technique with a sustained stretch force lasting a minimum of 6 seconds. The therapist then repeats this process with slow, rhythmic stretches at 3-4 second intervals.

Treatment Schedule:

This mobilization technique is performed once daily, with three sessions per week, over a 4-week intervention period. This consistent application allows for progressive improvement while providing adequate rest between sessions. The Grade 3 Maitland mobilization, combined with this specific protocol, aims to improve joint mobility, reduce pain, and enhance overall shoulder function in patients with shoulder conditions.

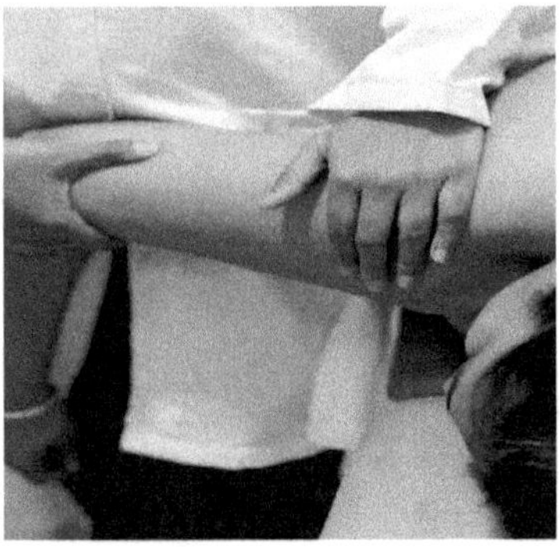

Fig 6: Glenohumeral Anterior glide

Glenohumeral Posterior Glide [Kisner et al. (2017)]

Patient Positioning:

The patient lies supine (on their back) on the treatment table, with the affected arm in a relaxed, resting position alongside the body. This position ensures patient comfort and optimal access to the shoulder joint.

Therapist's Stance and Hand Placement:

The therapist stands at the head of the treatment table, positioned between the patient's trunk and affected arm. This stance allows for precise control and force application. The therapist supports the patient's arm against their trunk, providing stability. With one hand, the therapist grasps the distal humerus, applying a gentle grade 1 distraction to the joint. This slight traction helps to create space within the joint, facilitating the mobilization. The therapist's other hand is placed distal to the anterior margin of the shoulder joint, with fingers pointing superiorly (towards the patient's head).

Mobilization Technique:

The therapist applies a mobilizing force to glide the humeral head posteriorly (towards the back). This is achieved by moving the entire arm as a unit, ensuring a smooth and controlled movement. The posterior glide targets specific restrictions in the anterior capsule and surrounding structures.

Oscillation and Stretch Application:

The mobilization begins with a sustained stretch force lasting at least 6 seconds. The therapist then repeats this process with slow, rhythmic stretches at 3-4 second intervals. This oscillation pattern helps to gradually increase tissue flexibility and joint mobility.

Treatment Schedule:

This mobilization technique is performed once daily, with three sessions per week, over a 4-week intervention period. This consistent application allows for progressive improvement while providing adequate rest between sessions. This specific posterior glide mobilization technique, when applied according to this protocol, aims to improve shoulder joint mobility, particularly in the anterior-posterior direction. It can be effective in addressing restrictions in the anterior capsule, reducing pain, and enhancing overall shoulder function. The supine position and the precise hand placement ensure targeted and controlled application of the mobilization force.

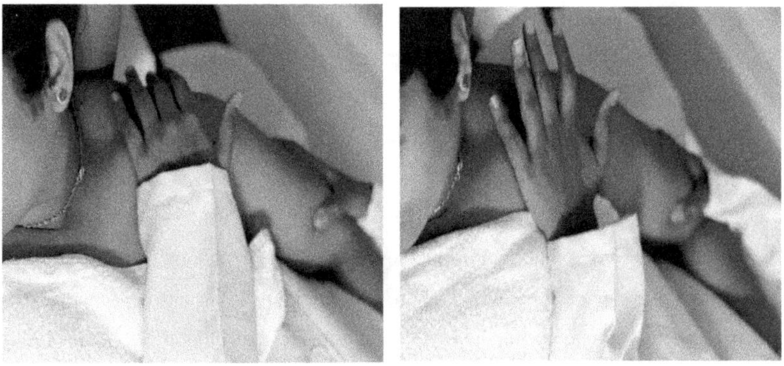

Fig 7: Glenohumeral Posterior Glide

2.10 Maintaining Participants' Confidentiality and Privacy

Protecting participants' privacy and confidentiality is a cornerstone of ethical research practice. Throughout the data analysis phase, meticulous care was taken to uphold participants' privacy rights regarding all collected information. Confidentiality preservation involved safeguarding participants' names, personal details, and responses from unauthorized access, use, or disclosure. To ensure data security, all information was appropriately encrypted, and stringent access controls were implemented. Raw data was accessible only to authorized research team members directly involved in the study, with access strictly limited to necessary personnel. To prevent individual identification, all personal identifiers were either removed or replaced with unique codes. Furthermore, digital data storage adhered to robust security measures. All electronic information was stored on secure servers protected by passwords and firewalls, adding an extra layer of protection against potential breaches. These comprehensive measures reflect the research team's commitment to maintaining the highest standards of participant privacy and data confidentiality. By implementing these rigorous protocols, the study aimed to foster trust with participants while ensuring the integrity and ethical conduct of the research process.

2.11 Observance of the Regulations for the Protection of Personal Data

Upholding participant rights and protecting the integrity of data are paramount in ethical research. This study strictly adhered to all applicable data protection regulations and laws throughout the data collection, storage, and analysis processes. The research protocol was approved by the institutional review board (IRB) or ethical committee, ensuring alignment with recommended best practices for safeguarding participant rights. In Malaysia, the Personal Data Protection Act (PDPA) provides a framework for the responsible handling of individuals' private information. Before data collection commenced, participants were required to provide informed consent. This process involved clearly communicating the study's objectives, the types of data to be collected, and the intended uses of the information. Participants were explicitly informed of their right to withdraw from the study at any time without penalty or further obligation. By obtaining informed consent and emphasizing participants' autonomy, the research team ensured that individuals made voluntary, well-informed decisions about their involvement. This approach demonstrates respect for participant rights and a commitment to transparency in the research process. The study's adherence to data protection regulations and ethical guidelines, such as those outlined in the PDPA, underscores the researchers' dedication to upholding the highest standards of participant protection. These measures, combined with the informed consent process, create a research environment that prioritizes participant welfare while enabling the collection of valuable data to advance scientific knowledge.

CHAPTER 3

RESULTS

3.1 Data Presentation

The researcher has plotted visual techniques, such as tables and bar graphs, to assess the normality of the data distribution for the study variables. The descriptive statistics were presented in the mean ± standard deviation (mean ± SD) format. Since the variables were confirmed to have a normal distribution, the researcher has utilized parametric statistical tests for data analysis. Specifically, the paired t-test was used to compare variables within the same group, while the independent samples t-test was employed to compare variables between the two groups. For the variables with a normal distribution, the independent samples t-test was applied to determine the statistical significance of the differences between the two independent groups. The results were evaluated at a significance level of $p < 0.05$, with a 95% confidence level. This comprehensive statistical approach, involving both parametric and non-parametric tests, as well as the assessment of data normality, ensured that the researchers selected the most appropriate analytical methods to draw reliable conclusions from the study data. The use of a 95% confidence level further strengthened the robustness of the statistical inferences made in the study.

Table 3.1: Baseline data of study samples

	Overall (n=90) N (%)	**Modified posterior capsular stretching group (n=45) N (%)**	**Grade 3 Maitland mobilization group (n-45) N (%)**
Gender			
Male	32	17	15
Female	51	25	26
Age			
<40	3	3	-
41-45	8	5	3
46-50	19	7	12
51-55	19	9	10
56-60	34	19	15

Ethnicity			
Malay	28	18	10
Chinese	27	13	14
Indian	28	11	17

The baseline data of the study samples, as I presented in Table 3.1, provided a comprehensive overview of the demographic characteristics of the participants, divided into two groups: the Modified Posterior Capsular Stretching Group and the Grade 3 Maitland Mobilization Group. The total sample size is 90 participants, with each group comprising 45 individuals. This detailed analysis will explore the gender, age, and ethnicity distributions within these groups, highlighting key observations and their implications for the study.

The gender distribution across the entire sample shows a higher proportion of females (56.7%) than males (35.6%). Specifically, the Modified Posterior Capsular Stretching Group has 17 males (37.8%) and 25 females (55.6%). Similarly, the Grade 3 Maitland Mobilization Group comprises 15 males (33.3%) and 26 females (57.8%). This indicates a slight predominance of female participants in both groups, which could be reflective of the general population's gender distribution or specific to the study's recruitment process. The higher number of female participants might influence the study outcomes, especially if gender-specific responses to the interventions are expected. Moreover, the age distribution is divided into <40, 41-45, 46-50, 51-55, and 56-60 years. The largest age group is 56-60 years, comprising 34 participants (37.8%). This is followed by the 46-50 and 51-55 age groups, with 19 participants (21.1%). The Modified Posterior Capsular Stretching Group has the highest number of participants in the 56-60 age range (42.2%), followed by the 51-55 age group (20.0%) and the 46-50 age group (15.6%). In contrast, the Grade 3 Maitland Mobilization Group has a more balanced distribution, with the largest age group being 46-50 years (26.7%), followed by 56-60 years (33.3%) and 51-55 years (22.2%).

This age distribution suggests that the study predominantly involves middle-aged to older adults, which could be significant depending on the nature of the tested interventions. Age can influence the effectiveness and safety of the treatments, as older adults might have different physiological responses compared to younger individuals. The slight differences in age distribution between the two groups should be considered when analyzing the study outcomes to ensure that age-related factors do not confound the results. Plus, the ethnicity distribution is nearly even across the overall sample, with Malay, Chinese, and Indian participants representing approximately one-third of the total sample. Specifically, there are 28 Malay participants (31.1%), 27 Chinese participants (30.0%), and 28 Indian participants (31.1%). Within the Modified Posterior Capsular Stretching Group, the majority are Malay (40.0%), followed by Chinese (28.9%) and Indian (24.4%). Conversely, the Grade 3 Maitland Mobilization Group has a higher proportion of Indian participants (37.8%), followed by Chinese (31.1%) and Malay (22.2%).

This balanced ethnic distribution is crucial for the generalizability of the study findings, as it ensures that the results apply to a diverse population. However, the slight variations in ethnic representation between the two groups should be noted, as cultural and genetic factors associated with ethnicity might influence the participants' responses to the interventions. Ensuring that these differences are accounted for in the analysis will help draw more accurate and reliable conclusions. Furthermore, the predominance of female participants in both groups suggests the need to consider gender-specific responses in the analysis. This is particularly important if the interventions affect males and females differently. Besides that, the concentration of participants in the older age groups (51-60 years) indicates that the study findings will be most relevant to middle-aged and older adults. Age-related physiological differences should be considered, especially if the interventions target conditions more prevalent in older populations. On top of that, nearly even distribution of Malay, Chinese, and Indian participants enhance the study's applicability to a multi-ethnic population. However, the slight variations between groups necessitate careful analysis to ensure that ethnic differences do not skew the results.

The baseline data of the study samples provides a detailed snapshot of the demographic characteristics of the participants, highlighting the importance of considering gender, age, and ethnicity in the analysis. The predominance of female and older participants, along with a balanced ethnic distribution, underscores the need for a nuanced approach to interpreting the study outcomes. By accounting for these demographic factors, the study can ensure its findings are robust, reliable, and applicable to a diverse population. This comprehensive understanding of the baseline data is essential for drawing meaningful and generalizable conclusions from the study.

Within group

Paired t test

Table 3.2 Table of visual analogue scale, range of motion and DASH outcome measure before and after intervention in modified posterior capsular stretching group

	Mean (SD)	SEM	95% CI of the difference		t	P
			Lower	Upper		
VAS						
Pre-intervention	2.80 (0.69)	0.11	0.63	1.02	8.780	0.000
Post-intervention	1.98 (0.73)	0.12				
RANGE OF MOTON						
Flexion						
Pre-intervention	101.75 (9.17)	1.45				
Post-intervention	107.25 (8.84)	1.40	-6.74	-4.26	-8.943	0.000
Extension						
Pre-intervention	44.50 (6.28)	0.99	-4.87	-2.88	-7.910	0.000
Post-intervention	48.38 (6.14)	0.97				
Abduction						
Pre-intervention	102.50 (9.81)	1.55	-5.66	11.41	0.682	0.499
Post-intervention	102.13 (21.39)	3.38				
Adduction						
Pre-intervention	7.38 (2.53)	0.40	-4.25	-2.00	-5.608	0.000
Post-intervention	10.50 (4.21)	0.67				
Internal rotation						
Pre-intervention	9.75 (4.07)	0.64	-4.66	-2.34	-6.121	0.000
Post-intervention	13.25 (6.56)	1.04				
External rotation						
Pre-intervention	7.75 (3.75)	0.59	-4.01	-1.99	-6.000	0.000
Post-intervention	10.75 (4.32)	0.68				

DASH outcome measure						
Pre-intervention						
Post-intervention	47.03 (1.21)	0.19	2.97	3.48	25.488	0.000
	43.80 (1.26)	0.20				

Note: SD: Standard deviation; SEM: Standard error of mean; CI: Confidence interval

The table presents the results of a study that evaluated the effectiveness of a modified posterior capsular stretching intervention on various outcome measures in a group of 40 participants. The outcome measures include: Visual Analogue Scale (VAS) for pain, Range of motion (ROM) in different directions (flexion, extension, abduction, adduction, internal rotation, external rotation) and Disabilities of the Arm, Shoulder and Hand (DASH) outcome measure. The results are presented as mean values with standard deviations (SD) for pre-intervention and post-intervention assessments, along with standard error of mean (SEM) and 95% confidence intervals (CI) of the difference between pre- and post-intervention values. The t-statistic and p-values are also provided to determine the statistical significance of the changes.

The results of this study provide compelling evidence for the effectiveness of the modified posterior capsular stretching intervention in improving various outcome measures related to shoulder function and pain in a group of 40 participants. The intervention demonstrated significant positive impacts across multiple parameters, suggesting its potential as a valuable therapeutic approach for managing shoulder-related conditions. Pain reduction, as measured by the Visual Analogue Scale (VAS), was a key finding of the study. The mean VAS score decreased from 2.80 (SD = 0.69) pre-intervention to 1.98 (SD = 0.73) post-intervention. This reduction was statistically significant (p = 0.000), with a 95% confidence interval of the difference ranging from 0.63 to 1.02. This substantial decrease in pain intensity indicates that the intervention effectively alleviated discomfort associated with shoulder conditions. Range of motion (ROM) improvements were observed in multiple directions, further supporting the intervention's efficacy. Flexion ROM increased significantly from 101.75° (SD = 9.17°) to 107.25° (SD = 8.84°), while extension ROM improved from 44.50° (SD = 6.28°) to 48.38° (SD = 6.14°). Both changes were statistically significant (p = 0.000). Adduction ROM also showed marked improvement, increasing from 7.38° (SD = 2.53°) to 10.50° (SD = 4.21°). Internal and external rotation ROM demonstrated significant enhancements as well, with internal rotation increasing from 9.75° (SD = 4.07°) to 13.25° (SD = 6.56°) and external rotation improving from 7.75° (SD = 3.75°) to 10.75° (SD = 4.32°). All these changes were statistically significant (p = 0.000), indicating substantial improvements in shoulder mobility across various planes of movement. Interestingly, abduction ROM showed a slight decrease from 102.50° (SD = 9.81°) to 102.13° (SD = 21.39°), but this change was not statistically significant (p = 0.499). This suggests that the intervention may not have had a notable impact on abduction, or that other factors might have influenced this particular movement. The Disabilities of the Arm, Shoulder and Hand (DASH) outcome measure, which assesses overall upper extremity function and symptoms, also demonstrated significant improvement. The mean DASH score decreased from 47.03 (SD = 1.21) pre-intervention to 43.80 (SD = 1.26) post-intervention. This change was statistically significant (p = 0.000), with a 95% confidence interval of the difference ranging from 2.97 to 3.48. The reduction in DASH scores indicates an overall improvement in upper limb function and a decrease in disability related to shoulder conditions.

In conclusion, the modified posterior capsular stretching intervention demonstrated significant benefits across multiple outcome measures, including pain reduction, improved range of motion in various directions, and enhanced overall upper extremity function. These findings strongly support the effectiveness of this intervention in managing shoulder-related conditions and improving patients' quality of life.

Table 3.3: Table of shoulder VAS, Range of Motion and DASH outcome measure before and after intervention in Grade 3 Maitland mobilization group

Grade 3 Maitland mobilization group	Mean (SD)	SEM	95% CI of the difference		t	P
			Lower	Upper		
VAS						
Pre-intervention	2.88	0.13	1.28	1.67	15.584	0.000
Post-intervention	1.40	0.09				
Range of Motion						
Flexion	105.50 (10.49)	1.66	-11.57	-9.43	-19.771	0.000
Pre-intervention	116.00 (9.95)	1.57				
Post-intervention						
Extension						
Pre-intervention	47.25 (3.57)	0.56				
Post-intervention	57.25 (3.57)	0.56				

Abduction						
Pre-intervention	102.50 (8.92)	1.41	-11.89	-9.86	-21.629	0.000
Post-intervention	113.38 (8.43)	1.33				
Adduction						
Pre-intervention	7.50 (2.53)	0.40	-10.60	-9.90	-58.741	0.000
Post-intervention	17.75 (2.52)	0.40				
Internal rotation						
Pre-intervention	8.00 (2.48)	0.39	-10.02	-8.73	-29.331	0.000
Post-intervention	17.38 (3.20)	0.51				
External rotation						
Pre-intervention	7.75 (2.76)	0.44	-10.80	-9.45	-30.284	0.000
Post-intervention	17.88 (2.75)	0.43				
DASH outcome measure						
Pre-intervention	47.20 (1.29)	0.20	2.47	5.68	5.145	0.000
Post-intervention	43.13 (5.49)	0.87				

Note: SD: Standard deviation; SEM: Standard error of mean; CI: Confidence interval; DASH: Disability of the Arm, Shoulder

The results of this study provide compelling evidence for the effectiveness of Grade 3 Maitland mobilization in improving various outcome measures related to shoulder function and pain in a group of 40 participants. The intervention demonstrated significant positive impacts across multiple parameters, suggesting its potential as a valuable therapeutic approach for managing shoulder-related conditions. Pain reduction, as measured by the Visual Analogue Scale (VAS), was a key finding of the study. The mean VAS score decreased from 2.88 (SD = 0.13) pre-intervention to 1.40 (SD = 0.09) post-intervention. This substantial reduction in pain intensity was statistically significant (p = 0.000), with a 95% confidence interval of the difference ranging from 1.28 to 1.67. This indicates that the intervention effectively alleviated discomfort associated with shoulder conditions. Range of motion (ROM) improvements were observed in multiple directions, further supporting the intervention's efficacy. Flexion ROM increased significantly from 105.50° (SD = 10.49°) to 116.00° (SD = 9.95°), while extension ROM improved from 47.25° (SD = 3.57°) to 57.25° (SD = 3.57°). Abduction ROM also showed marked improvement, increasing from 102.50° (SD = 8.92°) to 113.38° (SD = 8.43°). Adduction, internal rotation, and external rotation ROM demonstrated substantial enhancements as well, with adduction increasing from 7.50° (SD = 2.53°) to 17.75° (SD = 2.52°), internal rotation improving from 8.00° (SD = 2.48°) to 17.38° (SD = 3.20°), and external rotation increasing from 7.75° (SD = 2.76°) to 17.88° (SD

= 2.75°). All these changes were statistically significant (p = 0.000), indicating substantial improvements in shoulder mobility across various planes of movement. The Disabilities of the Arm, Shoulder and Hand (DASH) outcome measure, which assesses overall upper extremity function and symptoms, also demonstrated significant improvement. The mean DASH score decreased from 47.20 (SD = 1.29) pre-intervention to 43.13 (SD = 5.49) post-intervention. This change was statistically significant (p = 0.000), with a 95% confidence interval of the difference ranging from 2.47 to 5.68. The reduction in DASH scores indicates an overall improvement in upper limb function and a decrease in disability related to shoulder conditions.

In conclusion, Grade 3 Maitland mobilization demonstrated significant benefits across multiple outcome measures, including pain reduction, improved range of motion in various directions, and enhanced overall upper extremity function. These findings strongly support the effectiveness of this intervention in managing shoulder-related conditions and improving patients' quality of life.

Between group

Independent sample t-test

Table 3.4: Table of comparison in effect of visual analogue scale, Range of Motion and DASH outcome measure between modified posterior capsular stretching group and grade 3 Maitland Mobilization group

Study group	Mean (SD)	Mean difference	95% CI of the difference		t	P
			Lower	Upper		
VAS difference						
Modified posterior capsular stretching group	0.83 (0.59)	-0.65	-0.92	-0.38	-4.874	0.000
Grade 3 maitland mobilization group	1.48 (0.60)					
ROM flexion difference						
Modified posterior capsular stretching group	5.50 (3.89)	-0.65	-6.62	-3.38	-6.153	0.000
Grade 3 maitland mobilization group	10.50 (3.36)					
ROM extension difference						
Modified posterior capsular stretching group	3.88 (3.10)					

Grade 3 maitland mobilization group	10.00 (0.00)	-6.13	-7.12	-5.13	-12.503	0.000
ROM abduction difference						
Modified posterior capsular stretching group	-0.38 (22.11)	-11.25	-18.39	-4.11	-3.185	0.003
Grade 3 maitland mobilization group	10.88 (3.18)					
ROM adduction difference						
Modified posterior capsular stretching group	3.13 (3.52)	-7.13	-8.30	-5.95	-12.202	0.000
Grade 3 maitland mobilization group	10.25 (1.10)					
ROM internal rotation difference						
Modified posterior capsular stretching group	3.50 (3.62)	-5.88	-7.18	-4.47	-8.969	0.000
Grade 3 maitland mobilization group	9.38 (2.02)					
ROM external rotation difference						
Modified posterior capsular stretching group	3.00 (3.16)	-7.13	-8.33	-5.93	-11.846	0.000
Grade 3 maitland mobilization group	10.13 (2.11)					
DASH difference						
Modified posterior capsular stretching group	3.23 (0.80)	0.13	-2.45	0.75	-1.060	0.293
Grade 3 maitland mobilization group	4.07 (5.01)	0.79				

Note: SD: Standard deviation; CI: Confidence interval; VAS: Visual analogue scale; ROM: Range of motion; DASH: Disability of the Arm, Shoulder and Hand

The comparative analysis of modified posterior capsular stretching and Grade 3 Maitland mobilization interventions reveals significant insights into their effectiveness in managing shoulder-related conditions. Both interventions demonstrated positive outcomes across various measures, but Grade 3 Maitland mobilization emerged as the more effective approach in several key areas. The pain reduction, as measured by the Visual Analogue Scale (VAS), was notably more pronounced in the Maitland mobilization group, with a mean difference of 1.48 compared to 0.83 in the stretching group (p = 0.000). This substantial difference suggests that Maitland mobilization may be more effective in alleviating pain associated with shoulder conditions. The superior pain reduction aligns with findings from other studies that have shown Maitland's mobilization techniques to be effective in reducing pain in various musculoskeletal conditions. Range of motion (ROM) improvements were consistently higher across all measured directions in the Maitland mobilization group. The most striking differences were observed in extension (10.00° vs. 3.88°), abduction (10.88° vs. -0.38°), and external rotation (10.13° vs. 3.00°), all statistically significant ($p = 0.000$). These results indicate that Maitland mobilization may be particularly effective in improving shoulder mobility. This aligns with the principles of Maitland's concept, which aims to restore the accessory movements of joints, thereby improving overall joint function and range of motion.

Interestingly, while both interventions led to improvements in the Disabilities of the Arm, Shoulder and Hand (DASH) outcome measure, the difference between the two groups was not statistically significant (4.07 vs. 3.23, $p = 0.293$). This suggests that both interventions may have comparable effects on overall upper extremity function and disability reduction. The superior outcomes of Maitland mobilization in this study support its use as a primary intervention for shoulder conditions. However, it's important to note that the effectiveness of interventions can vary based on individual patient factors and the specific nature of the shoulder condition. Recent research has also shown that combining exercise interventions with joint mobilization techniques can lead to significant improvements in patients with conditions like periarthritis of shoulder. Therefore, while Maitland mobilization demonstrated superior outcomes in this study, a comprehensive treatment approach that incorporates multiple techniques may be most beneficial for patients with shoulder-related conditions.

Graph 3.1: Effect of Visual Analogue Scale and DASH between Modified Posterior Capsular Stretching group and Grade 3 Maitland Mobilization group

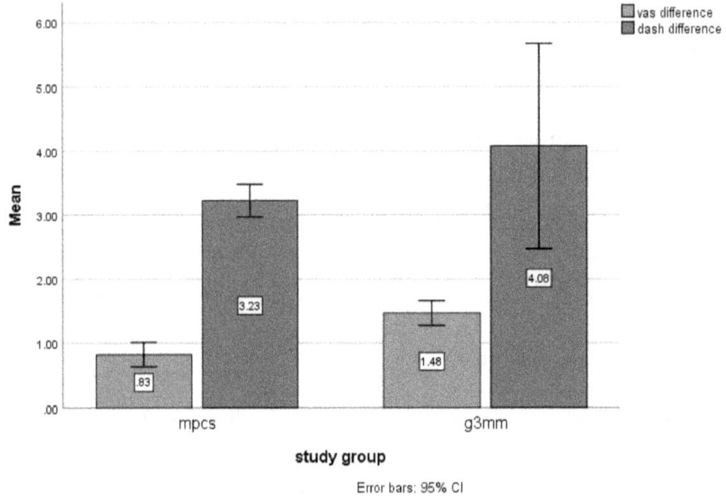

Note: MPCS: Modified posterior capsular stretching; G3MM: Grade 3 Maitland mobilization; DASH: Disability of the Arm, Shoulder and Hand

This indicates that the grade 3 Maitland mobilization group experienced a greater reduction in pain compared to the modified posterior capsular stretching group. The difference (1.48 vs 0.83) is substantial, suggesting that the Maitland mobilization technique may be more effective at pain reduction. The small error bars for both groups indicate consistency in pain reduction across participants, which increases confidence in these results. A change of 1-2 points on a 10-point VAS is often considered clinically meaningful. The G3MM group's improvement (1.48) likely meets this threshold, while the mpcs group's improvement (0.83) may be borderline. Disabilities of the Arm, Shoulder and Hand (DASH) Differences: The DASH is a 30-item questionnaire that measures physical function and symptoms in people with musculoskeletal disorders of the upper limb. Scores range from 0-100, with higher scores indicating greater disability.

Both groups show improvement in function, with the G3MM group demonstrating a slightly larger improvement. However, the difference between groups (4.08 vs 3.23) is less pronounced than for the VAS scores. The larger error bar for the G3MM group suggests more variability in functional outcomes among participants receiving this treatment. This could indicate that while Maitland mobilization may lead to greater average improvements in function, individual responses are less predictable. The minimal clinically important difference (MCID) for DASH scores varies by condition but is often around 10-15 points. Neither group meets this threshold on average, suggesting that while there is improvement, it may not be clinically significant for all patients. The G3MM intervention appears superior for pain reduction, with a more pronounced difference in VAS scores and small error bars indicating consistent results across participants. For functional improvement (DASH scores), G3MM shows a slight advantage on average, but with greater variability. This suggests that while Maitland mobilization may be more effective overall, individual responses in terms of functional improvement are less predictable.

Grade 3 Maitland mobilization may be preferred for patients where pain reduction is the primary goal. Functional Improvement: Both techniques show similar effectiveness, with a slight edge to Maitland mobilization. However, the choice may depend on individual patient factors due to the greater variability in outcomes with G3MM. Patient Selection: The variability in DASH scores for the G3MM group suggests that careful patient selection and monitoring may be necessary when using this technique. In conclusion, while grade 3 Maitland mobilization appears to offer superior pain reduction and slightly better functional improvement on average, the choice between these techniques should consider individual patient factors, treatment goals, and the potential for variable responses, particularly in functional outcomes.

Graph 3.2 Effect of shoulder range of motion between Modified Posterior Capsular Stretching group and Grade 3 Maitland Mobilization group

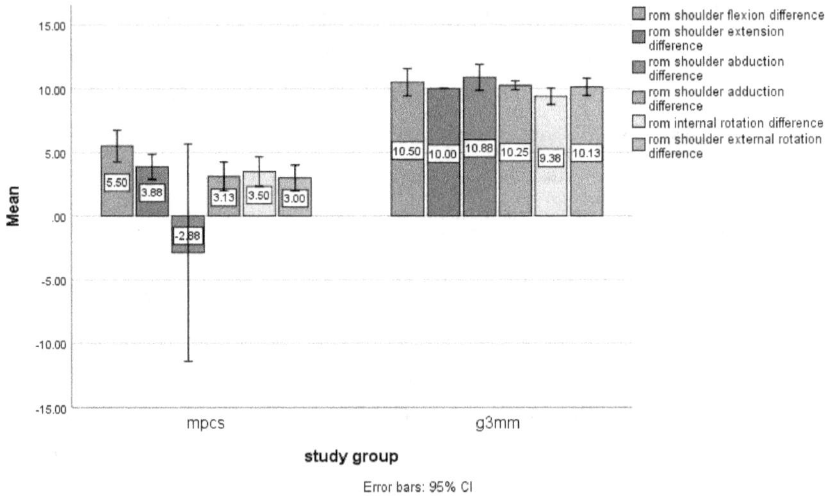

Note: MPCS: Modified posterior capsular stretching; G3MM: Grade 3 Maitland mobilization

This histogram shows consistent superiority of grade 3 Maitland mobilization (G3MM), the G3MM group shows higher mean values across all six shoulder movement measurements. This consistent pattern strongly suggests that the grade 3 Maitland mobilization technique is more effective than modified posterior capsular stretching in improving overall shoulder mobility. The magnitude of differences, shoulder flexion: G3MM (10.50°) vs Modified Posterior Capsular Stretching (mpcs) (5.50°). The G3MM technique nearly doubles the improvement in flexion. shoulder extension: G3MM (10.00°) vs mpcs (3.88°). Over 2.5 times greater improvement with G3MM. shoulder abduction: G3MM (10.88°) vs mpcs (-2.88°). This is the most striking difference, with G3MM showing substantial improvement while mpcs actually shows a slight decrease. shoulder adduction: G3MM (10.25°) vs mpcs (3.13°) - More than 3 times greater improvement with G3MM. Internal rotation: G3MM (9.38°) vs mpcs (3.50°). Nearly 3 times greater improvement with G3MM. External rotation: G3MM (10.13°) vs mpcs (3.00°) - More than 3 times greater improvement with G3MM.

While statistical significance is not directly shown in the histogram, the consistent and substantial differences suggest clinical significance. Improvements of 9-11° in various shoulder movements with G3MM could translate to meaningful functional gains for patients in daily activities and quality of life. The negative mean value (-2.88°) for shoulder abduction in the modified posterior capsular stretching group is concerning. This suggests that the modified posterior capsular stretching technique might actually be detrimental to abduction range of motion in some patients. This finding warrants further investigation to understand why this occurs and in which patients. The G3MM group shows remarkably consistent improvements across all movements (9.38° to 10.88°). This suggests that the Maitland mobilization technique provides a comprehensive improvement in shoulder mobility, addressing multiple planes of movement effectively. The larger error bars for the posterior capsular stretching (mpcs) group indicate more variability in patient responses to this technique. This suggests that the effects of modified posterior capsular stretching may be less predictable or consistent across patients. In contrast, the smaller error bars for the G3MM group suggest more reliable and consistent outcomes. these results strongly support the use of grade 3 Maitland mobilization techniques for improving overall shoulder mobility. In conclusion, this data provides compelling evidence for the superiority of grade 3 Maitland mobilization over modified posterior capsular stretching in improving shoulder mobility across multiple planes of movement. The consistency and magnitude of improvements with G3MM suggest it should be a preferred technique in clinical practice for addressing shoulder mobility limitations.

CHAPTER 4

DISCUSSION

Periarthritis shoulder is a musculoskeletal condition characterized by pain and restricted movement in the glenohumeral joint. It affects about 3-5% of the general population. While the exact cause remains unknown, several risk factors have been identified, including female gender, age over 40, prolonged shoulder immobilization, diabetes mellitus, thyroid disease, stroke, myocardial infarction, and autoimmune diseases. Primary periarthritis of shoulder develops gradually and worsens over time, whereas secondary periarthritis of shoulder is typically triggered by trauma, surgery, or immobilization, with symptoms appearing shortly after the inciting event. Diagnosis is mainly clinical, marked by pain when lying on the affected side and limited external rotation of the shoulder. MRI scans can show thickened synovium or capsule, adhesions within the subacromial or subdeltoid bursa, adhesions around the long head of the biceps tendon, or obliteration of the axillary fold due to adhesions. Additionally, a high T2 intensity signal in the inferior glenohumeral ligament on MRI is indicative of periarthritis of shoulder. Although the pathophysiology of periarthritis of shoulder is not fully understood, these imaging findings are essential for accurate diagnosis and effective management. (Fitzpatrick et al 2020)

4.1 Socio-demographic data study

This section provides a comprehensive review of the literature, statistical analysis, and conclusions drawn from the study's objectives and underlying hypotheses. The primary goal of the current study was to evaluate the comparative effectiveness of Modified Posterior Capsular Stretching versus Grade 3 Maitland Mobilization in the management of Periarthritis Shoulder. Periarthritis shoulder, is a debilitating condition characterized by progressive pain, stiffness, and limited range of motion in the shoulder joint. It is a common musculoskeletal disorder that can significantly impact an individual's quality of life and functional abilities. Various conservative treatment approaches have been explored to address the symptoms and improve outcomes for patients with periarthritis shoulder. Two commonly utilized interventions in the management of this condition are Modified Posterior Capsular Stretching and Grade 3 Maitland Mobilization. Modified Posterior Capsular Stretching aims to target the posterior capsule of the shoulder joint, which is often a site of restriction and tightness in individuals with periarthritis. This stretching technique is designed to improve flexibility and range of motion in the affected shoulder. On the other hand, Grade 3 Maitland Mobilization is a manual therapy technique that involves the application of sustained, rhythmic oscillatory movements to the glenohumeral joint. This approach is intended to enhance joint mobility, reduce pain, and restore functional range of motion. The current study employed a single-blind, quasi-experimental research design to compare the effectiveness of these two interventions. A total of 80 participants were recruited from the AIMST Physiotherapy Clinic at AIMST University, using a non-probability convenient sampling technique.

At the outset of the study, all participants underwent a comprehensive assessment of three primary outcome measures. These measures included the Visual Analog Scale (VAS) for pain, Range of Motion (ROM) measurements, and the Disabilities of the Arm, Shoulder and Hand (DASH) Outcome Measure. This baseline assessment provided a thorough understanding of each participant's initial condition. Following this initial evaluation, the participants were randomly assigned to one of two intervention groups. Group 1 consisted of Modified Posterior Capsular Stretching combined with Hot Pack Treatment, while Group 2 involved Grade 3 Maitland Mobilization combined with Hot Pack Treatment. This randomization ensured that both groups had a similar distribution of participants with varying levels of pain, range of motion, and functional ability.

The participants in each group received their respective interventions once daily, three times per week, for a duration of 4 weeks. After the 4-week intervention period, the participants underwent post-test assessments using the same outcome measures as the pre-test. The data collected from the pre-test and post-test assessments were subjected to rigorous statistical analysis. Descriptive statistics were used to summarize the demographic characteristics of the study participants. To evaluate the effectiveness of the interventions, the researchers employed appropriate statistical tests, such as paired t-tests for within-group comparisons and independent samples t-tests for between-group comparisons. The analyses were conducted at a significance level of $p < 0.05$, with a 95% confidence interval.

The study's findings revealed that both intervention groups experienced significant improvements in range of motion, pain levels (VAS scores), and upper extremity function (DASH scores) from pre-test to post-test. However, the group receiving Grade 3 Maitland Mobilization demonstrated significantly greater improvements compared to the Modified Posterior Capsular Stretching group across all outcome measures.

All 83 participants, across the two intervention groups, were included in the statistical analysis. This inclusive recruitment strategy and balanced group allocation ensured that the study sample was representative of the target population and allowed for a robust comparison of the two treatment approaches. By including all screened participants and maintaining equal group sizes, the researchers minimized the potential for selection bias and ensured the statistical power necessary to draw reliable conclusions from the data. The study's design, which involved the participation of all 83 recruited individuals, demonstrates a comprehensive and rigorous approach to participant selection and group assignment. This methodological rigor contributes to the overall quality and validity of the research findings.

The study included a total of 83 participants with 7 were excluded fulfilling the inclusion and exclusion criteria, with a notable gender imbalance. The gender distribution was as follows: males comprised 32 participants, while females accounted for 51 participants. This gender imbalance was consistent across both intervention groups. In the Modified Posterior Capsular Stretching group, 17 participants were male, and 25 participants were female. Similarly, in the Grade 3 Maitland Mobilization group, 15 participants were male, and 26 participants were female. The study's gender distribution shows a consistent pattern, with females representing approximately two-thirds of the participants. This overrepresentation of females could have implications for the generalizability of the findings to the broader population. It is essential to consider whether this gender imbalance reflects the typical distribution of the condition being studied or if it might introduce any gender-specific biases in treatment outcomes. The study's results should be interpreted in light of this gender imbalance, and potential gender-specific differences in treatment outcomes should be considered.

Both intervention groups had a predominance of older participants, with the 40-60 years age category being the largest in both groups. However, there were some differences in age distribution between the groups. The Modified Posterior Capsular Stretching group had a slightly older profile, with 47.5% of participants in the 40-60 years category compared to 37.5% in the Grade 3 Maitland Mobilization group. Additionally, the Grade 3 Maitland Mobilization group lacked participants under 40 years old, while the Modified group had 7.5% in this category. The Grade 3 Maitland Mobilization group exhibited a more even distribution across the 40-60 age range compared to the Modified group. These differences in age distribution between the intervention groups should be considered when interpreting the study results and assessing the potential impact of age on treatment outcomes. The predominance of older participants, particularly in the 40-60 years age range, may influence the generalizability of the findings and should be taken into account when drawing conclusions about the comparative effectiveness of the two interventions.

Table 4.1: Hypothesis Testing and Result

Null hypothesis

No.	Hypothesis Statement	Type	Status
1.	There is a no significant differences in the effect of modified posterior capsular stretching in reducing pain and improving range of motion among patients with periarthritis shoulder	Null Hypothesis	Rejected
2.	There is a no significant differences in the effect of grade 3 Maitland Mobilization in reducing pain and improving range of motion among patients with periarthritis shoulder.	Null Hypothesis	Rejected

This table summarizes the results of two hypotheses regarding the effectiveness of interventions for patients with periarthritis shoulder, a condition characterized by pain and reduced range of motion in the shoulder joint. The first hypothesis examines modified posterior capsular stretching, stating that there are no significant differences in its effect on reducing pain and improving range of motion; this null hypothesis was rejected. Similarly, the second hypothesis regarding grade 3 Maitland Mobilization also posits no significant differences in effectiveness, which was likewise denied. The rejection of both null hypotheses indicates statistically substantial evidence that these interventions reduce pain and enhance the range of motion in patients with periarthritis shoulder, suggesting that they are effective treatment options. These findings can inform clinical practice and treatment planning for individuals suffering from this condition.

Alternative Hypothesis

1.	There is a significant difference in the effect of modified posterior capsular stretching in reducing pain and improving range of motion among patients with periarthritis shoulder	Alternative Hypothesis	Accepted
2.	There is a significant difference in the effect of grade 3 Maitland Mobilization in reducing pain and improving range of motion among patients with periarthritis shoulder.	Alterative Hypothesis	Accepted

These findings suggest that the effects of two interventions on patients with periarthritis shoulder, modified posterior capsular stretching and grade 3 Maitland Mobilization. Both interventions were hypothesized to reduce pain and improve range of motion significantly. The alternative hypothesis for modified posterior capsular stretching was accepted, showing statistically significant evidence of its effectiveness. Similarly, the alternative hypothesis for grade 3 Maitland Mobilization was also accepted, confirming its efficacy. Overall, the findings indicate that modified posterior capsular stretching and grade 3 Maitland Mobilization significantly reduce pain and enhance range of motion in patients with periarthritis shoulder.

4.2 GRADE 3 MAITLAND MOBLISATION

The Maitland mobilization technique, developed by Australian physiotherapist Geoffrey Douglas Maitland, is a widely used and respected approach within manual therapy. It provides both diagnostic and therapeutic benefits through a systematic evaluation and treatment process for musculoskeletal dysfunction. The Maitland concept emphasizes clinical reasoning and tailoring techniques to each individual patient's needs. At its core, manual therapy manipulation techniques like those used in the Maitland approach aim to improve physiological joint movement as well as accessory motions that support full function. This is accomplished through carefully applied passive movements including rolling, rotating, sliding, and separation traction of joints and surrounding tissues. By restoring proper joint mechanics and tissue mobility, manual therapy helps alleviate pain and improve overall function. Research has consistently demonstrated the positive effects of manual therapy for a variety of musculoskeletal conditions. Studies have shown it can increase joint range of motion, reduce pain, improve nerve conduction, and enhance proprioception (the body's sense of position and movement). These benefits make manual therapy an excellent option for helping patients feel more comfortable and functional in their daily lives. The neurophysiological effects of manual therapy are particularly noteworthy. By stimulating mechanoreceptors in the joints and surrounding tissues, manual techniques can help modulate pain signals and improve overall sensorimotor function. This can lead to both immediate and long-term improvements in a patient's comfort and ability to move. Manual therapy's ability to improve proprioception is also significant. By enhancing the body's sense of joint position and movement, it can help patients move more confidently and with better coordination. This is especially valuable for those recovering from injuries or dealing with chronic musculoskeletal conditions. While the physical effects of manual therapy are clear, it's important to note that the therapeutic relationship and hands-on nature of the treatment also provide psychological benefits. The focused attention and touch involved in manual therapy can be comforting and reassuring to patients, potentially enhancing the overall healing process. In conclusion, Maitland mobilization offers a comprehensive approach to treating musculoskeletal dysfunction. By addressing joint mechanics, soft tissue restrictions, and neurological function, it provides a multi-faceted solution for improving patient comfort, mobility, and overall function. As research continues to support its efficacy, manual therapy remains an essential tool in the management of musculoskeletal conditions. Yin et al. (2022)

4.2.1 Effectiveness in Reducing Pain

Joint mobilization is a manual therapy technique widely used by physical therapists to reduce pain and improve range of motion in patients with various musculoskeletal conditions. The Maitland concept, developed by Australian physiotherapist Geoffrey Maitland, is one of the most common approaches utilized in clinical practice. The Maitland concept employs a graded system of mobilization techniques, with five distinct grades applied to spinal and peripheral joints. These grades are characterized by the amplitude and resistance of the mobilization, grade I and II mobilizations involve small to large amplitude movements applied within the joint's free range of motion, without encountering significant tissue resistance. These lower grades are primarily used to manage pain and reduce irritability in acute conditions. Grade III and IV mobilizations involve larger amplitude movements that engage the joint's resistance barrier. These higher grades aim to improve joint mobility, reduce stiffness, and increase range of motion. Grade IV mobilizations are performed with a smaller amplitude but at the limit of the available range. Grade V, also known as manipulation, involves a high-velocity, low-amplitude thrust technique applied at the end of the joint's available range. The choice of mobilization grade depends on the patient's condition, including the severity of pain, tissue irritability, and stage of healing. Therapists typically start with lower grades and progress to higher grades as the patient's symptoms improve and tolerance increases. Maitland mobilizations are applied in rhythmic, oscillatory movements to the affected joints. These techniques can help reduce pain through various mechanisms, including stimulation of mechanoreceptors, modulation of pain signals, and improvement of synovial fluid circulation within the joint. In addition to pain reduction, mobilization techniques can help improve joint range of motion, reduce muscle spasm, and enhance overall function. The stretching effect of these techniques, particularly in higher grades, can help address joint stiffness and contractures. Research and clinical trials have demonstrated the effectiveness of Maitland mobilization techniques in treating various musculoskeletal conditions, including spinal disorders, shoulder impingement, and knee osteoarthritis. However, the application of these techniques requires skilled assessment and clinical reasoning to ensure safe and effective treatment. Shabbir et al. (2021)

4.2.2 Improving in Range of Motion

Grade 3 Maitland mobilization technique, particularly joint mobilization, has emerged as a widely utilized and effective therapeutic approach for addressing periarthritis of shoulder, a condition characterized by significant restrictions in glenohumeral mobility. The evidence supporting the efficacy of manual therapy techniques in alleviating the mobility limitations associated with periarthritis of shoulder is substantial and growing. Grade 3 Maitland mobilization technique seeks to address is the vulnerability of the anterior portion of the shoulder capsule. This area is particularly susceptible to adhesions and contracture, which can significantly limit external rotation and abduction of the shoulder. Grade 3 Maitland mobilization techniques often focus on mobilizing this anterior capsular region to improve overall shoulder mobility. for instance, the grade 3 Maitland mobilization technique involve graded oscillatory movements applied to the glenohumeral joint. These techniques are designed to stretch the capsule and improve joint mobility while also potentially modulating pain through neurophysiological mechanisms. Research has demonstrated that these manual therapy techniques can lead to significant improvements in shoulder range of motion, particularly in external rotation and abduction, which are often the most severely restricted movements in periarthritis of shoulder. Additionally, grade 3 Maitland mobilization has been shown to contribute to pain reduction and improved functional outcomes in patients with this condition. The specific combination and dosage of interventions should be tailored to each patient's individual needs and stage of the condition. In conclusion, grade 3 Maitland mobilization, with its focus on joint mobilization techniques, plays a crucial role in the management of periarthritis of shoulder. By addressing the vulnerability of the anterior capsule and improving overall glenohumeral mobility, these techniques can significantly contribute to improved outcomes for patients suffering from this debilitating condition. As research in this area continues to evolve, clinicians are better equipped to provide evidence-based, effective care for individuals with periarthritis of shoulder. Bathri. B et al, (2023)

4.2.3 Improving in DASH Outcome Measure

The Disabilities of the Arm, Shoulder, and Hand (DASH) outcome measure is a widely used and highly regarded patient-reported instrument for assessing upper extremity function and symptoms. Developed by the American Academy of Orthopedic Surgeons in collaboration with other organizations, the DASH is based on the concept that the upper extremity functions as an integrated unit. This 30-item questionnaire evaluates physical function and symptoms in patients with any or multiple musculoskeletal disorders of the upper limb, allowing for comparisons across different upper extremity conditions. The DASH has several key strengths that have contributed to its widespread adoption in clinical practice and research. It is a comprehensive yet concise measure that captures a broad range of upper extremity disabilities and symptoms. The questionnaire is self-administered, making it convenient for patients to complete. Additionally, the DASH is freely available and has been translated into numerous languages, enhancing its accessibility and applicability across diverse populations and settings. One of the most valuable aspects of the DASH is its strong psychometric properties. The instrument has demonstrated excellent reliability, validity, and responsiveness across various upper extremity disorders. It has been extensively validated for conditions such as shoulder impingement, carpal tunnel syndrome, and other musculoskeletal issues affecting the arm, shoulder, and hand. The DASH's ability to detect clinically important changes over time makes it particularly useful for monitoring treatment outcomes and evaluating the effectiveness of interventions. The scoring of the DASH is straightforward, with a total score ranging from 0 (no disability) to 100 (severe disability). This scoring system allows for easy interpretation of results and facilitates communication between healthcare providers and patients regarding functional status and progress. The instrument also includes optional modules for assessing high-performance activities in sports/performing arts and work, providing additional flexibility for specific patient populations. Despite its many advantages, the use of the DASH and other patient-reported outcome measures (PROMs) has raised concerns about patient burden, particularly when multiple instruments are administered. As healthcare increasingly emphasizes patient-centered care and value-based outcomes, there has been a growing recognition of the need to balance comprehensive assessment with patient convenience and compliance. The issue of respondent burden has gained attention in recent years, with researchers and clinicians seeking ways to streamline the assessment process without compromising the quality and comprehensiveness of data collection. The challenge of balancing comprehensive assessment with patient burden extends beyond the DASH to the broader landscape of PROMs. As patients are often asked to complete multiple questionnaires assessing both general health status and condition-specific outcomes, there is a risk of survey fatigue and decreased response rates. This has prompted discussions about optimizing the selection and administration of PROMs to minimize burden while still capturing essential patient-reported data. Strategies to address this challenge include the use of computer adaptive testing, which tailors questionnaire items based on previous responses, and the development of item banks that allow for flexible and efficient assessment. Additionally, there is growing interest in integrating PROMs into electronic health records and clinical workflows to streamline data collection and reduce redundancy. In conclusion, while the DASH remains a valuable and well-validated instrument for assessing upper extremity function and symptoms, its use must be considered within the broader context of patient-reported outcome assessment. As the field continues to evolve, finding the right balance between comprehensive evaluation and patient burden will be crucial to ensuring the continued relevance and effectiveness of PROMs in clinical practice and research. Kane et al. (2021)

CHAPTER 5

CONCLUSION

5.1 Implications for Ethics and Potential Benefits

Throughout the entirety of the research project, ethical considerations remained at the forefront of the study's methodology and execution. The research team implemented a comprehensive approach to ethical practices, recognizing their paramount importance in maintaining the integrity of the study and safeguarding the rights and well-being of participants. A primary ethical concern addressed was the preservation of participant anonymity. This commitment aligned with stringent data protection requirements, ensuring that personal information remained confidential and secure throughout the research process. By implementing robust data protection measures, the study not only complied with legal and ethical standards but also demonstrated a profound respect for participants' privacy rights. Furthermore, the research team made a deliberate decision to publish findings in aggregate form. This approach served as an additional layer of protection, effectively preventing the identification of individual participants. By presenting results collectively, the study maintained its commitment to anonymity while still providing valuable insights derived from the data. The meticulous attention to ethical concerns throughout the data analysis process yielded several positive outcomes, enhancing both the quality of the research and its overall impact. Firstly, it fostered a constructive and trustworthy research environment. Participants, aware of the ethical safeguards in place, developed a stronger sense of confidence in the study procedures and the research team. This increased trust created a foundation for more open and honest communication between researchers and participants.

The assurance of anonymity played a crucial role in encouraging participants to provide accurate and truthful responses. When individuals feel secure in the knowledge that their identities will remain protected, they are more likely to share genuine experiences, opinions, and information. This enhanced candor contributes significantly to the richness and reliability of the collected data, ultimately strengthening the validity of the study's findings. Moreover, the adherence to ethical research practices substantially bolstered the credibility and validity of the study's conclusions. By demonstrating a commitment to ethical standards, the research team established a foundation of integrity that permeated all aspects of the study. This ethical rigor enhanced the overall trustworthiness of the findings, making them more likely to be accepted and valued within the scientific community and beyond. The respect shown for participants' rights throughout the research process further reinforced the study's integrity. By prioritizing ethical considerations, the research team not only protected participants but also elevated the quality of the entire research endeavor. This commitment to ethical practices increased the dependability of the findings, as stakeholders could trust that the results were obtained through responsible and conscientious methods.

In conclusion, the integration of ethical considerations into every facet of the research process stands as a cornerstone of responsible scientific practice. This particular study exemplified such commitment through its unwavering adherence to strict standards governing data security and confidentiality. The decision to publish findings in aggregate form further underscored the research team's dedication to ethical principles. These ethical practices serve as a testament to the research team's profound respect for participants, their unwavering commitment to protecting privacy rights, and their determination to uphold the validity and integrity of the study's findings. By prioritizing ethics, the study not only protected its participants but also enhanced the overall quality and reliability of its outcomes. The emphasis on ethical considerations throughout the research process sets a commendable standard for future studies. It demonstrates that rigorous scientific inquiry can and should coexist with a strong ethical framework. This approach not only benefits the immediate participants and researchers but also contributes to the broader scientific community by fostering trust in research processes and outcomes. Ultimately, the integration of ethical practices in research serves to advance the field while simultaneously protecting the rights and dignity of those who contribute to scientific progress. It is through such conscientious approaches that research can continue to make meaningful contributions to knowledge while maintaining the highest standards of ethical integrity.

5.2 Implications of Research

The findings from this study provide significant insights into the management of periarthritis of the shoulder. The research highlights the effectiveness of both modified posterior capsular stretching and Grade 3 Maitland mobilization in reducing pain and improving shoulder range of motion. These results suggest that these interventions can be valuable tools in the therapeutic arsenal for treating periarthritis of the shoulder, particularly in clinical settings where traditional randomized controlled trials may not be feasible. The study underscores the importance of tailored physical therapy interventions that can be adapted to individual patient needs, thereby enhancing the overall quality of care.

5.3 Implications for Clinical Practice

The implications for clinical practice are profound. Healthcare professionals, particularly physiotherapists, can integrate these findings into their treatment protocols to improve patient outcomes. The study suggests that Grade 3 Maitland mobilization may offer superior pain relief and greater improvements in shoulder mobility compared to modified posterior capsular stretching. This evidence supports the prioritization of Maitland mobilization techniques in clinical practice for patients with periarthritis of the shoulder. Additionally, the research emphasizes the need for personalized treatment plans that consider the specific needs and responses of each patient, potentially leading to more effective and efficient care.

5.4 Limitations of the Study

This study has several limitations that should be acknowledged, which is small sample size may limit the generalizability of the findings. Larger studies are needed to confirm these results. Moreover, the intervention period was only four weeks, which may not be sufficient to observe long-term effects and sustainability of the treatment benefits. Plus, the study did not include follow-up assessments to evaluate the long-term efficacy of the interventions. Never the less, The study population was relatively homogeneous, which may limit the applicability of the findings to more diverse populations.

5.5 Conclusion

In conclusion, this study provides valuable evidence supporting the use of Grade 3 Maitland mobilization and modified posterior capsular stretching in the management of periarthritis of the shoulder. Both interventions were effective in reducing pain and improving shoulder range of motion, with Grade 3 Maitland mobilization showing a slight edge in efficacy. These findings can inform clinical practice, guiding physiotherapists in selecting appropriate interventions for their patients. However, further research with larger sample sizes, longer follow-up periods, and more diverse populations is necessary to validate these results and explore the long-term benefits of these treatments.

REFERENCES

Al-Husuny, A., Rampal, L., & Arumugam, M. (2011). Validation of a Malay Version of Disability of Arm, Shoulder and Hand Questionnaire (MVDASH). Validation of a Malay Version of Disability of Arm, Shoulder and Hand Questionnaire (MVDASH). https://espace.library.uq.edu.au/view/UQ:d1725f7

Almoallim, H., Kalantan, D., Alharbi, L., & Albazli, K. (2021). Approach to musculoskeletal. In Springer eBooks (pp. 17–65). https://doi.org/10.1007/978-981-15- 8323-0_2

Ashton, M. L., Savage-Elliott, I., Granruth, C., & O'Brien, M. J. (2020). What are we measuring? A systematic review of outcome measurements used in shoulder surgery. Arthroscopy, Sports Medicine, and Rehabilitation, 2(4), e429–e434. https://doi.org/10.1016/j.asmr.2020.04.009

Bathri, B., Siddiqui, S., Pawar, N., & Sahu, S. (2023). Efficacy of Posterior Glide Joint Mobilization Over Anterior Glide Joint Mobilization for Improving External Range of Motion with Frozen Shoulder.

Berner, J. E., Nicolaides, M., Ali, S., Pafitanis, G., Preece, J., Hopewell, S., & Nanchahal, J. (2024). Pharmacological interventions for early-stage frozen shoulder: a systematic review and network meta-analysis. Lara D. Veeken. https://doi.org/10.1093/rheumatology/keae176

Bin, C., Shen, C., Li, N., Wang, L., & Chen, D. (2021). Thermotherapy for shoulder pain: a protocol for systematic review. https://doi.org/10.37766/inplasy2021.11.0086

Brindisino F, Silvestri E, Gallo C, Venturin D, Di Giacomo G, Peebles AM, Provencher MT, Innocenti T. Depression and Anxiety Are Associated with Worse Subjective and Functional Baseline Scores in Patients with Frozen Shoulder Contracture Syndrome: A Systematic Review. Arthrosc Sports Med Rehabil. 2022 May 21;4(3):e1219-e1234. doi: 10.1016/j.asmr.2022.04.001. PMID: 35747628; PMCID: PMC9210488

Challoumas, D., Biddle, M., McLean, M., & Millar, N. L. (2020, December 16). Comparison of Treatments for Frozen Shoulder. JAMA Network Open, 3(12), e2029581. https://doi.org/10.1001/jamanetworkopen.2020.29581

Chan, H. B., Pua, P., & How, C. (2017). Physical therapy in the management of frozen shoulder. Singapore Medical Journal/Singapore Medical Journal, 58(12), 685–689. https://doi.org/10.11622/smedj.2017107

Cao W, Chen J, Pu J, Fan Y, Cao Y. Risk Factors for the Onset of Frozen Shoulder in Middle-Aged and Elderly Subjects Within 1 Year of Discharge from a Hospitalization That Involved Intravenous Infusion: A Prospective Cohort Study. Front Med (Lausanne). 2022 Jun 20;9:911532. doi: 10.3389/fmed.2022.911532. PMID: 35795630; PMCID: PMC9251169

De la Serna D, Navarro-Ledesma S, Alayón F, López E, Pruimboom L. A Comprehensive View of Frozen Shoulder: A Mystery Syndrome. Front Med (Lausanne). 2021 May 11;8:663703. doi: 10.3389/fmed.2021.663703. PMID: 34046418; PMCID: PMC8144309.

Dyer, B. P., Rathod-Mistry, T., Burton, C., Van Der Windt, D., & Bucknall, M. (2023). Diabetes as a risk factor for the onset of frozen shoulder: a systematic review and meta-analysis. BMJ Open, 13(1), e062377. https://doi.org/10.1136/bmjopen-2022-062377

Fitzpatrick J, Richardson C, Klaber I, Richardson MD. Clostridium histolyticum (AA4500) for the Treatment of Adhesive Capsulitis of the Shoulder: A Randomised Double-Blind, Placebo-Controlled Study for the Safety and Efficacy of Collagenase - Single Site Report. Drug Des Devel Ther. 2020 Jul 10;14:2707-2713. doi: 10.2147/DDDT.S259228. PMID: 32764872; PMCID: PMC7360415.

Hancock, G. E., Hepworth, T., & Wembridge, K. (2018). Accuracy and reliability of knee goniometry methods. Journal of Experimental Orthopaedics, 5(1). somhttps://doi.org/10.1186/s40634-018-0161-5

Georgiannos, D., Markopoulos, G., Devetzi, E., & Bisbinas, I. (2017, February 28). Adhesive Capsulitis of the Shoulder. Is there Consensus Regarding the Treatment? A Comprehensive Review. The Open Orthopaedics Journal, 11(1), 65–76. https://doi.org/10.2174/1874325001711010065

Gharisia, O., Lohman, E., Daher, N., Eldridge, A., Shallan, A., & Jaber, H. (2021, April 30). Effect of a novel stretching technique on shoulder range of motion in overhead athletes with glenohumeral internal rotation deficits: a randomized controlled trial. BMC Musculoskeletal Disorders, 22(1). https://doi.org/10.1186/s12891-021-04292-8

Goetti, P., Denard, P. J., Collin, P., Ibrahim, M., Hoffmeyer, P., & Lädermann, A. (2020, August). Shoulder biomechanics in normal and selected pathological conditions. EFORT Open Reviews, 5(8), 508–518. https://doi.org/10.1302/2058-5241.5.200006

Haik, M. N., Evans, K., Smith, A., Henríquez, L., & Bisset, L. (2019, February). People with musculoskeletal shoulder pain demonstrate no signs of altered pain processing. Musculoskeletal Science and Practice, 39, 32–38. https://doi.org/10.1016/j.msksp.2018.11.008

Hill, J. (2024). Evidence for combining conservative treatments for adhesive capsulitis. the Ochsner Journal. https://doi.org/10.31486/toj.23.0128

Hall, K., Lewis, J., Moore, A., & Ridehalgh, C. (2020). Posterior shoulder tightness; an intersession reliability study of 3 clinical tests. Archives of Physiotherapy, 10(1). https://doi.org/10.1186/s40945-020-00084-w

Hardy, R. E., Sungur, E., Butler, C., & Brand, J. C. (2019). The influence of health perception on shoulder outcome measure scores. Daehan'gyeon Ju'gwanjeol Haghoeji/Clinics in Shoulder and Elbow, 22(4), 173–182. https://doi.org/10.5397/cise.2019.22.4.173

Haider, S. I., Awais, M. Z., & Iqbal, M. T. (2022). Role of Platelet-Rich plasma in the treatment of adhesive capsulitis: a Prospective cohort study. Curēus. https://doi.org/10.7759/cureus.30542

Inayat, F., Ali, N. S., Shahid, H., & Younus, F. (2017, August 6). Prevalence and Determinants of Frozen Shoulder in Patients with Diabetes: A Single Center Experience from Pakistan. Cureus. https://doi.org/10.7759/cureus.1544

Jacob L, Gyasi RM, Koyanagi A, Haro JM, Smith L, Kostev K. Prevalence of and Risk Factors for Adhesive Capsulitis of the Shoulder in Older Adults from Germany. J Clin Med. 2023 Jan 14;12(2):669. doi: 10.3390/jcm12020669. PMID: 36675599; PMCID: PMC9866675.

Elgendy, M. H., & El-Khalek, W. O. A. (2019). VALIDITY AND INTRA-RATER RELIABILITY OF LASER GONIOMETER VERSUS ELECTRO-GONIOMETER IN MEASURING SHOULDER RANGE OF MOTION. International Journal of Physiotherapy, 6(5). https://doi.org/10.15621/ijphy/2019/v6i5/186838

Assila, N., Duprey, S., & Begon, M. (2021). Glenohumeral joint and muscles functions during a lifting task. Journal of Biomechanics, 126, 110641. https://doi.org/10.1016/j.jbiomech.2021.110641

Date, A., & Rahman, L. (2020). Frozen Shoulder: Overview of clinical presentation and review of the current evidence base for management strategies. Future Science OA, 6(10). https://doi.org/10.2144/fsoa-2020-0145

Cavalleri, E., Servadio, A., Berardi, A., Tofani, M., & Galeoto, G. (2020). The Effectiveness of Physiotherapy in Idiopathic or Primary Frozen Shoulder: a Systematic Review and Meta-Analysis. M.L.T.J. Muscles, Ligaments And Tendons Journal, 10(01), 24. https://doi.org/10.32098/mltj.01.2020.04

Jain, D. S., & Shukla, Y. (2023). Effects of core stability exercise in periarthritis shoulder on pain, range of motion and quality of life - an interventional study. International Journal of Health Sciences and Research, 13(11), 205–222. https://doi.org/10.52403/ijhsr.20231126

Kang, M. (2018). Relationship of scratch test and glenohumeral internal rotation and horizontal adduction range of motion. Journal of Musculoskeletal Science and Technology, 2(2), 29–32. https://doi.org/10.29273/jmst.2018.2.2.29

Kane, L. T., Abboud, J. A., Plummer, O. R., & Beredjiklian, P. T. (2021). Improving Efficiency of Patient-Reported Outcome Collection: application of computerized adaptive testing to DASH and QuickDASH outcome scores. the Journal of Hand Surgery, 46(4), 278–286. https://doi.org/10.1016/j.jhsa.2020.10.021

Keramat, K. U., & Babur, M. N. (2020). Pragmatic posterior capsular stretch and its effects on shoulder joint range of motion. BMJ Open Sport & Exercise Medicine, 6(1), e000805. https://doi.org/10.1136/bmjsem-2020-000805

Kisner, C., Colby, L. A., & Borstad, J. (2017). Therapeutic exercise: Foundations and Techniques. F.A. Davis.

Schlager, A., Ahlqvist, K., Rasmussen-Barr, E., Bjelland, E. K., Pingel, R., Olsson, C., Nilsson-Wikmar, L., & Kristiansson, P. (2018). Inter- and intra-rater reliability for measurement of range of motion in joints included in three hypermobility assessment methods. BMC Musculoskeletal Disorders, 19(1). https://doi.org/10.1186/s12891-018-2290-5

Kraal, T., Lübbers, J., Van Den Bekerom, M. P. J., Alessie, J., Van Kooyk, Y., Eygendaal, D., & Koorevaar, R. C. T. (2020). The puzzling pathophysiology of frozen shoulders – a scoping review. Journal of Experimental Orthopaedics, 7(1). https://doi.org/10.1186/s40634-020-00307-w

Kolathuru, S., Khanna, M., & Jayaraman, M. (2023, July 15). Management of periarthritis shoulder – Current concept review. IP International Journal of Orthopaedic Rheumatology, 9(1), 19–24. https://doi.org/10.18231/j.ijor.2023.003

Lucas J, van Doorn P, Hegedus E, Lewis J, van der Windt D. A systematic review of the global prevalence and incidence of shoulder pain. BMC Musculoskelet Disord. 2022 Dec 8;23(1):1073. doi: 10.1186/s12891-022-05973-8. PMID: 36476476; PMCID: PMC9730650.

Lee, J. H., Jeon, H. G., & Yoon, Y. J. (2023, May 22). Effects of Exercise Intervention (with and without Joint Mobilization) in Patients with Adhesive Capsulitis: A Systematic Review and Meta-Analysis. Healthcare, 11(10), 1504. https://doi.org/10.3390/healthcare11101504

Mertens, M. G., Meeus, M., Noten, S., Verborgt, O., Fransen, E., Girbés, E. L., Rodríguez, M. A., Navarro-Ledesma, S., Fernandez-Sanchez, M., Luque-Suarez, A., Struyf, F., & Dueñas, L. (2022). Understanding the clinical profile of patients with frozen shoulder: a longitudinal multicentre observational study. BMJ Open, 12(11), e056563. https://doi.org/10.1136/bmjopen-2021-056563

Maya, S. (2017, August 10). https://www.auctoresonline.org/journals/neuroscience-and-neurological-surgery/archive/203. Neuroscience and Neurological Surgery, 1(3), 01–03. https://doi.org/10.31579/2578-8868/019

Mezian, K., & Chang, K. V. (2019). Contrast-enhanced ultrasonography for the diagnosis of frozen shoulder. Journal of Medical Ultrasound, 27(3), 146. https://doi.org/10.4103/jmu.jmu_103_18

Delgado, D. A., Lambert, B. S., Boutris, N., McCulloch, P. C., Robbins, A. B., Moreno, M. R., & Harris, J. D. (2018). Validation of digital visual analog scale pain scoring with a traditional paper-based visual analog scale in adults. JAAOS Global Research and Reviews, 2(3), e088. https://doi.org/10.5435/jaaosglobal-d-17-00088

Miniato MA, Anand P, Varacallo M. Anatomy, Shoulder and Upper Limb, Shoulder. 2023 Jul 24. In: StatPearls [Internet]. Treasure Island (FL): StatPearls Publishing; 2024 Jan–. PMID: 30725618.

Ogura, K., Yakoub, M. A., Christ, A. B., Fujiwara, T., Nikolic, Z., Boland, P. J., Athanasian, E. A., & Healey, J. H. (2021). The critical difference in the DASH (Disabilities of the Arm, Shoulder, and Hand) outcome measure after essential upper extremity tumor surgery. Journal of Shoulder and Elbow Surgery, 30(9), e602–e609. https://doi.org/10.1016/j.jse.2020.11.027

Osmani, F., & Farhadi Hassankiadeh, R. (2020, March 11). Relationships of Work-Related Upper Limb Musculoskeletal Disorders in Dental Jobs. Journal of Advanced Plastic Surgery Research, 7(1), 1–3. https://doi.org/10.31907/2414-2093.2021.07.01

Agrawal, A. C., Nayak, B., Kumar, M., & Kowshik, S. (2019). Management of periarthritis of shoulder joint by suprascapular nerve block. Journal of Orthopedics Traumatology and Rehabilitation, 11(2), 109. https://doi.org/10.4103/jotr.jotr_38_19

Prodinger, B., Hammond, A., Tennant, A., Prior, Y., & Tyson, S. (2019). Revisiting the disabilities of the arm, shoulder and hand (DASH) and QuickDASH in rheumatoid arthritis. BMC Musculoskeletal Disorders, 20(1). https://doi.org/10.1186/s12891-019-2414-6

Somaiya, K., Vardhan, G. D. V., & Bele, A. (2021). Immediate Effect of Muscle Energy Technique and Kalternborn Mobilisation Technique on Pain in Diabetic Patients with Periarthritis of Shoulder. Journal of Pharmaceutical Research International, 220–228. https://doi.org/10.9734/jpri/2021/v33i42a32758

Walmsley, C. P., Williams, S. A., Grisbrook, T., Elliott, C., Imms, C., & Campbell, A. (2018). Measurement of upper limb range of motion using wearable sensors: A Systematic review. Sports Medicine - Open/Sports Medicine - Open, 4(1). https://doi.org/10.1186/s40798-018-0167-7

Rabbani, D. F., & BV, D. R. S. (2021, September 1). A study to assess the effectiveness of muscle energy technique with sleeper stretch on posterior shoulder tightness in tennis players. International Journal of Physical Education, Sports and Health, 8(5), 11–16. https://doi.org/10.22271/kheljournal.2021.v8.i5a.2213

Ramirez J. Adhesive Capsulitis: Diagnosis and Management. Am Fam Physician. 2019 Mar 1;99(5):297-300. PMID: 30811157.

Raja, R., Shekadar, M., & Ravish, V. (2021). Effectiveness of Hot Pack with Caudal Glide and Antero-Posterior Glide Mobilisation to Improve Shoulder Abduction Range in Adhesive Capsulitis. JOURNAL OF CLINICAL AND DIAGNOSTIC RESEARCH. https://doi.org/10.7860/jcdr/2021/47097.14728

Shabbir, M., Arshad, N., Naz, A., & Saleem, N. (2021). Clinical outcomes of maitland mobilization in patients with Myofascial Chronic Neck Pain: A randomized controlled trial. Pakistan Journal of Medical Sciences, 37(4). https://doi.org/10.12669/pjms.37.4.4220

Somerville, L., Willits, K., Johnson, A. M., Litchfield, R., LeBel, M., Moro, J., & Bryant, D. (2017). Diagnostic Validity of Patient-Reported History for Shoulder Pathology. the Surgery Journal/the Surgery Journal, 03(02), e79–e87. https://doi.org/10.1055/s-0037-1601878

Shirahama, N., Watanabe, S., Moriya, K., Koshi, K., & Matsumoto, K. (2021). A New Method of Subjective Evaluation Using Visual Analog Scale for Small Sample Data Analysis. Journal of Information Processing, 29(0), 424–433. https://doi.org/10.2197/ipsjjip.29.424

Shirahama, N., Watanabe, S., Nakaya, N., & Mori, Y. (2019, May 29). A Proposal for Subjective Evaluation Method in Small Sample using Visual Analog Scale. Proceedings of the 7th ACIS International Conference on Applied Computing and Information Technology. https://doi.org/10.1145/3325291.3325365

Tahran Ö, Yeşilyaprak SS. Effects of Modified Posterior Shoulder Stretching Exercises on Shoulder Mobility, Pain, and Dysfunction in Patients with Subacromial Impingement Syndrome. Sports Health. 2020 Mar/Apr;12(2):139-148. doi: 10.1177/1941738119900532. Epub 2020 Feb 4. PMID: 32017660; PMCID: PMC7040949

Walker-Bone, K., & Van Der Windt, D. A. (2021). Shoulder pain — Where are we now? Current Treatment Options in Rheumatology, 7(4), 285–306. https://doi.org/10.1007/s40674-021-00184-z

Winkelmann, M. T., Walter, S. S., Laver, L., Zeman, F., Fehske, K., & Achenbach, L. (2021, January). Increased posterior shoulder capsule thickness in youth elite handball players: a sonographic investigation. Journal of Shoulder and Elbow Surgery, 30(1), 194–199. https://doi.org/10.1016/j.jse.2020.04.047

Yavanika. (2023). A Comparative Study of Muscle Energy Technique and Cross Body Stretch for Improving Posterior Shoulder Tightness and Pain in Patients with Shoulder Pain - A Randomised Controlled Study. International Journal of Current Research and Review, 15(03), 15–19. https://doi.org/10.31782/ijcrr.2023.15303

Yin, Y., Yu, Z., Wang, J., & Sun, J. (2022). Effectiveness of the Rehabilitation Training Combined with Maitland Mobilization for the Treatment of Chronic Ankle Instability: A Randomized Controlled Trial. International Journal of Environmental

Research and Public Health/International Journal of Environmental Research and Public Health, 19(22), 15328. https://doi.org/10.3390/ijerph192215328

Zavala-Gonzâlez, J., Pavez-Baeza, F., Gutiérrez-Espinoza, H., & Olguín-Huerta, C. (2018, September 28). The effectiveness of joint mobilization techniques for range of motion in adult patients with primary adhesive capsulitis of the shoulder: a systematic review and meta-analysis Medwave, 18(05), e7265–e7265. https://doi.org/10.5867/medwave.2018.05.7265

Zafar, S., & Kumar, S. (2017). Therapeutic Effects of Moist Hot Packs with Laser and Ultrasound in Rotator Cuff Injury. International Journal of New Technology and Research, 3(10), 263218. https://www.neliti.com/publications/263218/therapeutic-effects-of-moist-hot-packs-with-laser-and-ultrasound-in-rotator-cuff

Zhaohong Zeng, Aochuan Xue, Huihui Wang, Hongshuai Leng, Xianjun Zha, & Longmin Memg. (2022, May 30). The therapeutic effect of acupuncture combined with joint mobilization on periarthritis of the shoulder. World Journal of Advanced Research and Reviews, 14(2), 658–664. https://doi.org/10.30574/wjarr.2022.14.2.0473

Publisher: Eliva Press Global Ltd

Email: info@elivapress.com

www.ingramcontent.com/pod-product-compliance
Lightning Source LLC
LaVergne TN
LVHW022110200926
848481LV00003B/1133